THE ANTI INFLAMMATORY LIFESTYLE DIET:

" A Guide to Nourishing Your Body and Simple Meal Plan to Optimize Immunity"

OLIVIA BRENDA

TABLE OF CONTENTS

INTRODUCTION TO INFLAMMATION AND ITS IMPACT ON HEALTH

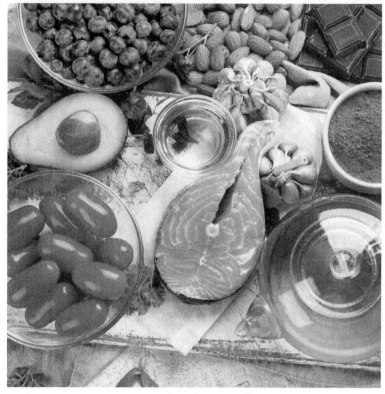

Inflammation is a natural and essential response of the body's immune system to injury, infection, or harmful stimuli. It serves as a protective mechanism to initiate the healing process and defend against foreign invaders. While acute inflammation is a necessary and temporary response, chronic inflammation can have detrimental effects on overall health and wellbeing.

Inflammation is a complex biological response involving various cells, chemicals, and signaling pathways. When tissues are damaged or infected, the immune system releases pro-inflammatory mediators, such as cytokines and chemokines, to recruit immune cells to the site of injury. This results in characteristic symptoms such as redness, swelling, heat, and pain, which are indicative of the body's attempt to repair and protect itself.

While acute inflammation is a short-term and localized response, chronic inflammation is a persistent and systemic condition that can contribute to the development and progression of numerous diseases. Research has shown that chronic inflammation plays a central role in the pathogenesis of conditions such as cardiovascular disease, type 2 diabetes, obesity, autoimmune disorders, neurodegenerative diseases, and certain cancers.

Given the significant impact of chronic inflammation on health outcomes, adopting an anti-inflammatory lifestyle is paramount for disease prevention and management. An anti-inflammatory lifestyle encompasses dietary choices, physical activity, stress management, adequate sleep, and other lifestyle factors that help mitigate inflammation and support overall wellbeing.

By understanding the underlying mechanisms of inflammation and its implications for health, individuals can make informed decisions to promote inflammation resolution and reduce the risk of chronic disease. This book will explore the principles of the anti-inflammatory diet, strategies for identifying and avoiding inflammatory triggers, practical tips for incorporating anti-inflammatory foods into your meals, and lifestyle modifications to support long-term inflammation management.

Through knowledge, empowerment, and actionable steps, readers will learn how to harness the power of an anti-inflammatory lifestyle to optimize their health and vitality, one meal and lifestyle choice at a time.

What is inflammation?

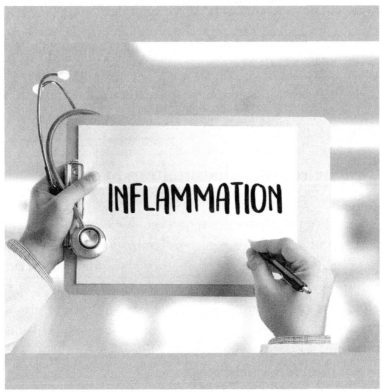

Inflammation is a complex biological response that occurs in the body when tissues are damaged, infected, or injured. It is a fundamental part of the immune system's defense mechanism and serves to protect the body from harmful stimuli, such as pathogens, toxins, or physical trauma. When inflammation occurs, the immune system releases various signaling molecules, including cytokines and chemokines, which attract immune cells to the affected area. This leads to characteristic symptoms such as redness, swelling, heat, and pain. The goal of inflammation is to remove the harmful stimuli and initiate the healing process, ultimately restoring tissue homeostasis and function. While acute inflammation is a normal and necessary response, chronic inflammation, which persists over time, can contribute to the development and progression of various diseases, including cardiovascular disease, diabetes, arthritis, and cancer.

The role of inflammation in chronic diseases

The role of inflammation in chronic diseases is significant and multifaceted. Chronic inflammation refers to a persistent, low-grade inflammatory state that can occur throughout the body, often without obvious symptoms. Unlike acute inflammation, which is a temporary and localized response to injury or infection, chronic inflammation can contribute to the development and progression of various diseases.

Cardiovascular Disease: Chronic inflammation plays a key role in the pathogenesis of cardiovascular diseases such as atherosclerosis, coronary artery disease, and stroke. Inflammatory processes contribute to the formation of plaques in the arteries, leading to narrowing and reduced blood flow. Additionally, inflammation can destabilize these plaques, increasing the risk of heart attacks and other cardiovascular events.

Type 2 Diabetes: Inflammation is closely linked to insulin resistance, a hallmark of type 2 diabetes. Chronic inflammation can impair insulin signaling pathways, leading to elevated blood sugar levels and insulin resistance. This inflammatory state can also contribute to pancreatic beta-cell dysfunction and further exacerbate glucose intolerance.

Obesity: Adipose tissue, or fat cells, produce pro-inflammatory cytokines and other molecules that contribute to chronic low-grade inflammation. This adipose tissue inflammation is thought to be a key factor in the development of obesity-related complications such as insulin resistance, metabolic syndrome, and cardiovascular disease.

Autoimmune Disorders: In autoimmune diseases such as rheumatoid arthritis, lupus, and multiple sclerosis, the immune system mistakenly attacks healthy tissues, leading to chronic inflammation and tissue damage. Inflammation is a central feature of these conditions and contributes to ongoing symptoms and disease progression.

Cancer: Chronic inflammation has been implicated in various stages of cancer development, including initiation, promotion, and metastasis. Inflammatory processes can create a microenvironment that promotes tumor growth, angiogenesis (formation of new blood vessels), and immune evasion. Chronic inflammation can also contribute to DNA damage and genomic instability, increasing the risk of cancerous mutations.

Overall, chronic inflammation is increasingly recognized as a common underlying factor in the development of many chronic diseases. Addressing inflammation through lifestyle modifications, including diet, exercise, stress management, and sleep, can play a crucial role in preventing and managing these conditions.

Why an anti-inflammatory lifestyle matters?

An anti-inflammatory lifestyle matters because chronic inflammation is increasingly recognized as a central contributor to the development and progression of various chronic diseases. By adopting habits and making choices that help to mitigate inflammation, individuals can support their overall health and reduce the risk of disease. Here are several reasons why an anti-inflammatory lifestyle is important:

Disease Prevention: Chronic inflammation is linked to a wide range of diseases, including cardiovascular disease, type 2 diabetes, obesity, autoimmune disorders, and certain cancers. By reducing inflammation, individuals can lower their risk of developing these conditions and promote long-term health and wellbeing.

Improved Immune Function: Chronic inflammation can compromise immune function, making individuals more susceptible to infections and other immune-related disorders. By adopting an anti-inflammatory lifestyle, individuals can support a balanced immune response and enhance their body's ability to fight off pathogens and maintain health.

Reduced Pain and Discomfort: Inflammation is often associated with pain, swelling, and discomfort, particularly in conditions such as arthritis and inflammatory bowel disease. By reducing inflammation through lifestyle changes, individuals may experience relief from symptoms and improve their quality of life.

Enhanced Heart Health: Chronic inflammation is a key factor in the development of cardiovascular disease, including atherosclerosis, coronary artery disease, and stroke. Adopting an anti-inflammatory lifestyle can help to protect against these conditions by reducing inflammation in the arteries and promoting heart health.

Optimized Weight Management: Inflammation is closely linked to obesity and metabolic syndrome, conditions characterized by chronic low-grade inflammation and insulin resistance. By following an anti-inflammatory diet and lifestyle, individuals can support weight management goals and improve metabolic health.

Better Mental Health: Emerging research suggests that chronic inflammation may contribute to mood disorders such as depression and anxiety. By reducing inflammation through diet, exercise, and stress management, individuals may experience improvements in mental health and emotional wellbeing.

Longevity and Vitality: By promoting overall health and reducing the risk of chronic disease, an anti-inflammatory lifestyle can contribute to increased longevity and vitality. By prioritizing habits that support inflammation resolution, individuals can enjoy a higher quality of life and maintain independence as they age.

Overall, an anti-inflammatory lifestyle offers numerous benefits for health and wellbeing, making it a valuable approach for disease prevention, symptom management, and overall vitality. By making informed choices and adopting habits that support inflammation reduction, individuals can take proactive steps to optimize their health and promote longevity.

UNDERSTANDING THE ANTI-INFLAMMATORY DIET

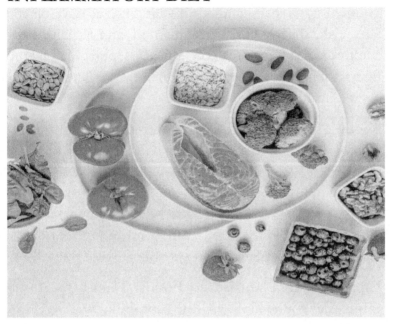

Understanding the Anti-Inflammatory Diet is crucial for anyone looking to optimize their health and reduce the risk of chronic disease. This dietary approach focuses on consuming foods that help to combat inflammation in the body while avoiding those that contribute to inflammation. Here's a breakdown of key points to consider:

Principles of the Anti-Inflammatory Diet: The anti-inflammatory diet emphasizes whole, nutrient-dense foods that are rich in antioxidants, vitamins, minerals, and other bioactive compounds. It encourages a balance of macronutrients, with an emphasis on healthy fats, lean proteins, and complex carbohydrates.

Key Components of an Anti-Inflammatory Diet: The diet includes plenty of fruits, vegetables, whole grains, legumes, nuts, seeds, and healthy fats such as olive oil and fatty fish. These foods are high in anti-inflammatory compounds such as omega-3 fatty acids, polyphenols, and fiber, which help to reduce inflammation and support overall health.

Foods to Avoid: The anti-inflammatory diet recommends minimizing or avoiding foods that are known to promote inflammation, such as refined carbohydrates, sugary snacks and beverages, processed meats, fried foods, and foods high in trans fats and saturated fats. These foods can contribute to oxidative stress, insulin resistance, and systemic inflammation.

Emphasis on Plant-Based Foods: Plant-based foods form the foundation of the anti-inflammatory diet, providing a wide range of nutrients and phytochemicals with anti-inflammatory properties. Eating a variety of colorful fruits and vegetables, whole grains, legumes, and nuts can help to reduce inflammation and support overall health.

Healthy Fats: Healthy fats, particularly those found in fatty fish, nuts, seeds, and olive oil, are an important part of the anti-inflammatory diet. These fats provide omega-3 fatty acids, which have potent anti-inflammatory effects and help to balance the body's inflammatory response.

Lean Proteins: Lean sources of protein, such as poultry, fish, tofu, legumes, and low-fat dairy products, are recommended on the anti-inflammatory diet. These protein sources provide essential amino acids for muscle repair and growth without contributing to inflammation.

Hydration: Adequate hydration is essential for overall health and inflammation management. Water is the best choice for hydration, but herbal teas and infused water can also be enjoyed as part of the anti-inflammatory diet.

By understanding and following the principles of the anti-inflammatory diet, individuals can make informed choices about the foods they eat to support inflammation reduction and promote optimal health and wellbeing. Incorporating a variety of nutrient-dense foods while minimizing processed and inflammatory foods can help to maintain a healthy balance and support long-term health goals.

Principles of the anti-inflammatory diet

The principles of the anti-inflammatory diet revolve around making food choices that help reduce inflammation in the body. Here are the key principles:

Emphasize Whole, Plant-Based Foods: The foundation of the anti-inflammatory diet consists of whole, minimally processed plant-based foods such as fruits, vegetables, whole grains, legumes, nuts, and seeds. These foods are rich in antioxidants, vitamins, minerals, and phytochemicals that help combat inflammation and support overall health.

Include Omega-3 Fatty Acids: Omega-3 fatty acids, found in fatty fish like salmon, mackerel, and sardines, as well as in walnuts, flaxseeds, and chia seeds, have potent anti-inflammatory properties. Including sources of omega-3s in the diet helps to balance the body's inflammatory response.

Opt for Healthy Fats: Choose healthy fats such as olive oil, avocado oil, nuts, and seeds over saturated and trans fats found in processed and fried foods. Healthy fats help reduce inflammation and support cardiovascular health.

Limit Processed and Refined Foods: Minimize consumption of processed foods, refined carbohydrates, sugary snacks, and beverages, as these can promote inflammation and contribute to chronic disease risk. Instead, focus on whole, nutrient-dense foods.

Choose Lean Proteins: Incorporate lean sources of protein such as poultry, fish, tofu, legumes, and low-fat dairy products into your meals. Protein is essential for muscle repair and growth, and choosing lean sources helps reduce intake of pro-inflammatory fats.

Eat a Variety of Colorful Fruits and Vegetables: Different colored fruits and vegetables contain a variety of phytochemicals with anti-inflammatory properties. Aim to include a rainbow of colors in your meals to maximize the diversity of nutrients and antioxidants.

Prioritize Fiber-Rich Foods: Fiber-rich foods such as fruits, vegetables, whole grains, legumes, and nuts help promote gut health and reduce inflammation. Fiber also helps regulate blood sugar levels and promotes satiety, aiding in weight management.

Stay Hydrated: Adequate hydration is essential for overall health and inflammation management. Drink plenty of water throughout the day and limit consumption of sugary beverages and alcohol, which can contribute to inflammation.

By following these principles, individuals can create a balanced and nutritious diet that helps reduce inflammation, supports overall health, and reduces the risk of chronic diseases associated with inflammation.

Key components of an anti-inflammatory diet

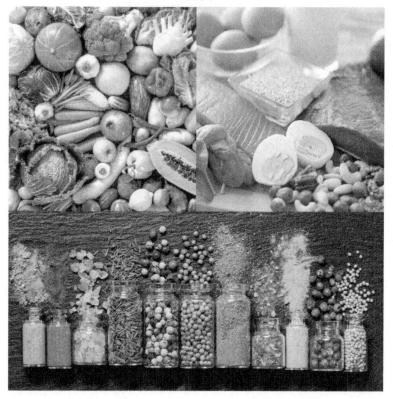

The key components of an anti-inflammatory diet encompass a variety of foods rich in nutrients and compounds that help reduce inflammation in the body while minimizing or avoiding those that promote inflammation. Here are the key components:

Fruits and Vegetables: Colorful fruits and vegetables are rich in antioxidants, vitamins, minerals, and phytochemicals that help combat inflammation. Aim to include a variety of fruits and vegetables in your diet, such as berries, leafy greens, cruciferous vegetables, tomatoes, peppers, and citrus fruits.

Whole Grains: Whole grains like brown rice, quinoa, oats, barley, and whole wheat provide fiber, vitamins, minerals, and antioxidants. These nutrients help regulate blood sugar levels, promote gut health, and reduce inflammation.

Healthy Fats: Choose sources of healthy fats such as oily fish (salmon, mackerel, sardines), nuts (almonds, walnuts), seeds (flaxseeds, chia seeds), avocado, and olive oil. These fats contain omega-3 fatty acids and monounsaturated fats, which have anti-inflammatory properties and support heart health.

Lean Proteins: Include lean sources of protein in your diet, such as poultry (chicken, turkey), fish, tofu, tempeh, legumes (beans, lentils), and low-fat dairy products. Protein is essential for muscle repair and growth, and choosing lean sources helps reduce intake of pro-inflammatory fats.

Herbs and Spices: Incorporate herbs and spices into your meals to add flavor and boost anti-inflammatory properties. Examples include turmeric, ginger, garlic, cinnamon, rosemary, and basil, which contain compounds with potent anti-inflammatory effects.

Probiotic-Rich Foods: Probiotics are beneficial bacteria that help promote gut health and reduce inflammation. Include fermented foods such as yogurt, kefir, kimchi, sauerkraut, and miso in your diet to support a healthy balance of gut bacteria.

Anti-Inflammatory Beverages: Stay hydrated with water and incorporate anti-inflammatory beverages such as green tea, herbal teas (ginger, chamomile), and fresh vegetable juices. These beverages provide hydration and additional antioxidants to combat inflammation.

Moderation of Red Meat and Processed Foods: While red meat and processed foods should be limited in an anti-inflammatory diet, they can still be enjoyed in moderation. Opt for lean cuts of red meat and minimize consumption of processed meats, sugary snacks, refined carbohydrates, and fried foods, which can promote inflammation and increase the risk of chronic diseases.

By including these key components in your diet and focusing on whole, nutrient-dense foods, you can create a balanced and anti-inflammatory eating pattern that supports overall health and wellbeing.

Benefits of adopting an anti-inflammatory diet

Adopting an anti-inflammatory diet offers a multitude of benefits for overall health and wellbeing. Here are some of the key benefits:

Reduced Inflammation: Perhaps the most significant benefit of adopting an anti-inflammatory diet is the reduction of chronic inflammation throughout the body. By consuming foods that help to combat inflammation and avoiding those that promote it, individuals can lower levels of pro-inflammatory markers in the blood and tissues, thereby reducing the risk of chronic diseases associated with inflammation.

Lower Risk of Chronic Disease: Chronic inflammation is a common underlying factor in the development of many chronic diseases, including cardiovascular disease, type 2 diabetes, obesity, autoimmune disorders, and certain cancers. By mitigating inflammation through dietary choices, individuals can lower their risk of developing these conditions and promote overall health and longevity.

Improved Heart Health: An anti-inflammatory diet supports heart health by reducing inflammation in the arteries and lowering the risk of atherosclerosis, coronary artery disease, and stroke. Consuming foods rich in omega-3 fatty acids, antioxidants, and fiber helps to lower cholesterol levels, regulate blood pressure, and improve endothelial function, all of which contribute to a healthier cardiovascular system.

Better Blood Sugar Control: The anti-inflammatory diet emphasizes whole, nutrient-dense foods that help regulate blood sugar levels and reduce insulin resistance. By avoiding refined carbohydrates and sugary snacks, individuals can stabilize blood glucose levels and lower the risk of developing type 2 diabetes and metabolic syndrome.

Weight Management: Adopting an anti-inflammatory diet can support weight management goals by promoting satiety, reducing cravings, and improving metabolic function. Whole, fiber-rich foods help to keep you feeling full and satisfied, while healthy fats and lean proteins provide sustained energy and support muscle mass.

Enhanced Gut Health: Many of the foods included in an anti-inflammatory diet, such as fruits, vegetables, whole grains, and fermented foods, promote a healthy balance of gut bacteria and support digestive health. This can lead to improved nutrient absorption, reduced inflammation in the gut, and a lower risk of gastrointestinal disorders such as irritable bowel syndrome (IBS) and inflammatory bowel disease (IBD).

Increased Energy and Vitality: Eating a diet rich in whole, nutrient-dense foods provides the body with the energy and nutrients it needs to function optimally. By fueling your body with nourishing foods and avoiding processed and inflammatory foods that can drain energy levels, you may experience increased vitality, mental clarity, and overall wellbeing.

Overall, adopting an anti-inflammatory diet offers numerous benefits for health and wellbeing, making it a valuable approach for disease prevention, symptom management, and overall vitality. By making informed choices about the foods you eat and prioritizing habits that support inflammation reduction, you can optimize your health and enhance your quality of life.

THE SCIENCE BEHIND INFLAMMATION: CAUSES AND EFFECTS

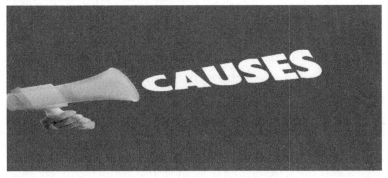

The science behind inflammation is complex and involves a coordinated response of the immune system to injury, infection, or tissue damage. Here's an overview of the key components and processes involved:

Initiation of Inflammation: Inflammation is triggered by various stimuli, including pathogens (such as bacteria, viruses, or fungi), physical injury, toxins, or autoimmune reactions. When tissues are damaged or threatened, immune cells release signaling molecules called cytokines, which act as messengers to initiate the inflammatory response.

Role of Immune Cells: Immune cells play a central role in the inflammatory process. Neutrophils are among the first responders to inflammation, migrating to the site of injury or infection to engulf and destroy pathogens. Macrophages are another type of immune cell that engulfs and digests pathogens, cellular debris, and foreign substances. These cells also release additional cytokines to recruit more immune cells to the site of inflammation.

Vasodilation and Increased Permeability: In response to cytokines and other inflammatory mediators, blood vessels in the affected area dilate and become more permeable. This allows immune cells, proteins, and fluid to move from the bloodstream into the surrounding tissue, leading to the characteristic symptoms of inflammation, such as redness, swelling, heat, and pain.

Release of Pro-inflammatory Mediators: In addition to cytokines, other pro-inflammatory mediators such as prostaglandins, leukotrienes, and histamine are released during inflammation. These molecules help amplify the inflammatory response, recruit more immune cells to the site of injury or infection, and promote tissue repair and healing.

Resolution of Inflammation: Inflammation is a tightly regulated process that is intended to be self-limiting. Once the threat has been neutralized and tissue repair is underway, anti-inflammatory mediators are released to dampen the inflammatory response and promote resolution. Specialized pro-resolving mediators (SPMs) help to switch off inflammation, clear debris, and restore tissue homeostasis.

Chronic Inflammation: While acute inflammation is a normal and necessary response to injury or infection, chronic inflammation occurs when the inflammatory response persists over time. Chronic inflammation can be triggered by factors such as persistent infection, autoimmune disorders, obesity, smoking, stress, or environmental toxins. Prolonged inflammation can damage healthy tissues and contribute to the development of chronic diseases such as cardiovascular disease, diabetes, arthritis, and cancer.

Understanding the science behind inflammation is crucial for developing strategies to modulate the inflammatory response and promote health and wellbeing. By targeting the underlying mechanisms of inflammation, researchers and healthcare professionals can develop novel therapies and interventions to treat and prevent inflammatory diseases.

Chronic inflammation vs. acute inflammation

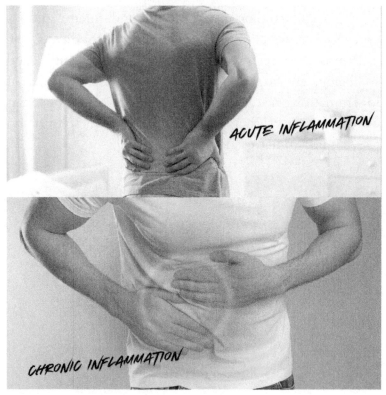

ACUTE INFLAMMATION

CHRONIC INFLAMMATION

Chronic inflammation and acute inflammation are two distinct types of inflammatory responses, each with different characteristics, causes, and effects:

Acute Inflammation:

- Duration: Acute inflammation is a short-term and self-limiting response that occurs rapidly in response to tissue injury, infection, or trauma. It typically resolves within a few days to weeks once the underlying trigger is removed or neutralized.

- Causes: Acute inflammation is triggered by various stimuli, including pathogens (such as bacteria, viruses, or fungi), physical injury, toxins, or autoimmune reactions.

- Symptoms: The hallmark symptoms of acute inflammation include redness, swelling, heat, pain, and loss of function at the site of injury or infection. These symptoms are localized to the affected area and are part of the body's natural defense mechanism to eliminate harmful stimuli and initiate tissue repair.

- Immune Response: Acute inflammation involves a rapid and coordinated response of the immune system, including the release of pro-inflammatory mediators such as cytokines, chemokines, and prostaglandins. Immune cells such as neutrophils and macrophages migrate to the site of inflammation to engulf and destroy pathogens, clear debris, and initiate tissue repair.

- Resolution: Acute inflammation is intended to be self-limiting and resolves once the threat has been neutralized and tissue repair is underway. Specialized pro-resolving mediators (SPMs) help to switch off inflammation, clear debris, and restore tissue homeostasis.

Chronic Inflammation:

- Duration: Chronic inflammation is a persistent and low-grade inflammatory state that can last for weeks, months, or even years. Unlike acute inflammation, which resolves quickly, chronic inflammation can persist even in the absence of an obvious trigger.

- Causes: Chronic inflammation can be triggered by factors such as persistent infection, autoimmune disorders, obesity, smoking, stress, environmental toxins, or long-term exposure to inflammatory dietary factors.
- Symptoms: The symptoms of chronic inflammation are often subtle and may not be as localized or pronounced as those of acute inflammation. Chronic inflammation can manifest as systemic symptoms such as fatigue, malaise, low-grade fever, and general feelings of unwellness.
- Immune Response: Chronic inflammation involves a dysregulated and prolonged immune response, characterized by persistent activation of pro-inflammatory pathways and inadequate resolution of inflammation. Over time, chronic inflammation can lead to tissue damage, fibrosis, and dysfunction.
- Consequences: Chronic inflammation is implicated in the pathogenesis of many chronic diseases, including cardiovascular disease, type 2 diabetes, obesity, autoimmune disorders, neurodegenerative diseases, and certain cancers. Prolonged exposure to inflammatory mediators can contribute to tissue damage, impaired healing, and systemic complications.

In summary, acute inflammation is a normal and necessary response to injury or infection, whereas chronic inflammation is a persistent and dysregulated inflammatory state associated with many chronic diseases. Understanding the differences between these two types of inflammation is crucial for developing targeted interventions to prevent and manage inflammatory conditions.

Triggers of inflammation in the body

Inflammation in the body can be triggered by a variety of factors, including:

Infections: Pathogens such as bacteria, viruses, fungi, and parasites can trigger an inflammatory response when they invade the body. The immune system detects the presence of these invaders and releases pro-inflammatory cytokines and other mediators to combat the infection.

Physical Injury: Trauma, burns, cuts, bruises, and other forms of physical injury can cause tissue damage, leading to inflammation. The body responds to tissue damage by initiating the inflammatory process to repair injured tissues and prevent infection.

Autoimmune Disorders: In autoimmune diseases, the immune system mistakenly attacks healthy tissues, leading to chronic inflammation and tissue damage. Conditions such as rheumatoid arthritis, lupus, and multiple sclerosis are examples of autoimmune disorders characterized by inflammation.

Environmental Factors: Exposure to environmental pollutants, toxins, allergens, and irritants can trigger inflammation in the body. Common environmental triggers include air pollution, cigarette smoke, industrial chemicals, pollen, dust mites, and mold.

Dietary Factors: Certain dietary factors can promote inflammation in the body. Diets high in processed foods, refined carbohydrates, sugary snacks, trans fats, and excessive alcohol consumption have been linked to increased inflammation. On the other hand, diets rich in whole, nutrient-dense foods such as fruits, vegetables, whole grains, and healthy fats can help reduce inflammation.

Chronic Stress: Prolonged or chronic stress can dysregulate the immune system and promote inflammation in the body. Stress hormones such as cortisol and adrenaline can trigger inflammatory pathways and suppress immune function, making individuals more susceptible to inflammation-related diseases.

Obesity: Adipose tissue, or fat cells, produce pro-inflammatory cytokines and other molecules that contribute to chronic low-grade inflammation. Obesity is associated with increased levels of inflammation in the body, which can contribute to the development of obesity-related complications such as insulin resistance, metabolic syndrome, and cardiovascular disease.

Sedentary Lifestyle: Lack of physical activity and a sedentary lifestyle have been linked to increased inflammation in the body. Regular exercise helps to reduce inflammation by improving circulation, reducing oxidative stress, and modulating inflammatory pathways.

By understanding the various triggers of inflammation, individuals can take proactive steps to minimize their exposure to inflammatory stimuli and promote inflammation resolution. Lifestyle modifications such as maintaining a healthy diet, managing stress, staying physically active, and avoiding environmental toxins can help support a balanced inflammatory response and overall health and wellbeing.

Health consequences of prolonged inflammation

Prolonged inflammation can have a wide range of health consequences, impacting various systems and organs in the body. Here are some of the potential health consequences of chronic inflammation:

Increased Risk of Chronic Diseases: Chronic inflammation is a common underlying factor in the development and progression of many chronic diseases. Conditions such as cardiovascular disease, type 2 diabetes, obesity, autoimmune disorders, neurodegenerative diseases, and certain cancers are associated with prolonged inflammation.

Cardiovascular Disease: Chronic inflammation is implicated in the pathogenesis of cardiovascular diseases such as atherosclerosis, coronary artery disease, and stroke. Inflammatory processes contribute to the formation of plaques in the arteries, leading to narrowing and reduced blood flow. Chronic inflammation can also destabilize these plaques, increasing the risk of heart attacks and other cardiovascular events.

Type 2 Diabetes and Metabolic Syndrome: Chronic inflammation is closely linked to insulin resistance, a hallmark of type 2 diabetes and metabolic syndrome. Inflammatory mediators can impair insulin signaling pathways, leading to elevated blood sugar levels and insulin resistance. Chronic inflammation also contributes to pancreatic beta-cell dysfunction and further exacerbates glucose intolerance.

Obesity and Metabolic Disorders: Adipose tissue, or fat cells, produce pro-inflammatory cytokines and other molecules that contribute to chronic low-grade inflammation. Obesity is associated with increased levels of inflammation in the body, which can contribute to the development of obesity-related complications such as insulin resistance, metabolic syndrome, fatty liver disease, and cardiovascular disease.

Autoimmune Disorders: Chronic inflammation plays a central role in the pathogenesis of autoimmune diseases such as rheumatoid arthritis, lupus, multiple sclerosis, and inflammatory bowel disease. In these conditions, the immune system mistakenly attacks healthy tissues, leading to chronic inflammation and tissue damage.

Neurodegenerative Diseases: Chronic inflammation has been implicated in the pathogenesis of neurodegenerative diseases such as Alzheimer's disease, Parkinson's disease, and multiple sclerosis. Inflammatory processes in the brain can contribute to neuronal damage, neuroinflammation, and cognitive decline.

Cancer: Prolonged inflammation is associated with an increased risk of certain cancers. Inflammatory processes can create a microenvironment that promotes tumor growth, angiogenesis (formation of new blood vessels), metastasis, and immune evasion. Chronic inflammation can also contribute to DNA damage and genomic instability, increasing the risk of cancerous mutations.

Impaired Immune Function: Chronic inflammation can compromise immune function, making individuals more susceptible to infections and other immune-related disorders. Inflammatory cytokines can disrupt immune cell function and impair the body's ability to fight off pathogens.

Overall, prolonged inflammation is a significant risk factor for many chronic diseases and can have detrimental effects on overall health and wellbeing. Addressing inflammation through lifestyle modifications, including diet, exercise, stress management, and sleep, is crucial for preventing and managing inflammation-related diseases and promoting optimal health and longevity.

IDENTIFYING INFLAMMATORY FOODS AND INGREDIENTS

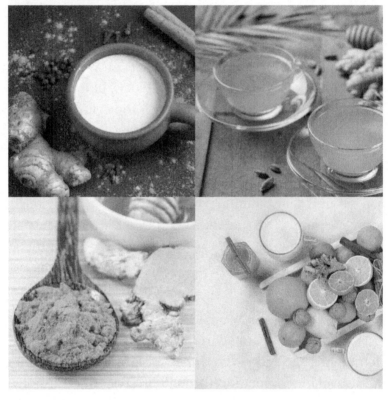

Identifying inflammatory foods and ingredients is an essential step in adopting an anti-inflammatory diet and reducing inflammation in the body. Here are some common inflammatory foods and ingredients to be aware of:

Refined Carbohydrates: Foods made with refined grains and sugars, such as white bread, white rice, sugary snacks, pastries, and desserts, can promote inflammation in the body. These foods have a high glycemic index, which can lead to spikes in blood sugar levels and contribute to insulin resistance and inflammation.

Processed Meats: Processed meats such as bacon, sausage, hot dogs, and deli meats often contain additives, preservatives, and high levels of saturated fats and sodium, all of which can promote inflammation and increase the risk of chronic diseases.

Trans Fats: Trans fats, also known as partially hydrogenated oils, are commonly found in processed and fried foods, margarine, shortening, and packaged snacks. These fats are highly inflammatory and have been linked to increased inflammation, insulin resistance, and cardiovascular disease risk.

Saturated Fats: While some sources of saturated fats, such as coconut oil and dairy products, may have neutral or even anti-inflammatory effects, excessive consumption of saturated fats from sources such as red meat, full-fat dairy, and butter can promote inflammation and increase the risk of chronic diseases.

Omega-6 Fatty Acids: Omega-6 fatty acids are essential fats found in vegetable oils such as soybean oil, corn oil, and sunflower oil. While omega-6 fatty acids are necessary for health, an imbalance between omega-6 and omega-3 fatty acids in the diet can promote inflammation. It's important to consume these fats in moderation and focus on increasing intake of omega-3 fatty acids from sources such as fatty fish, flaxseeds, and walnuts.

Artificial Additives and Preservatives: Many processed and packaged foods contain artificial additives, preservatives, flavorings, and colorings that can trigger inflammation in sensitive individuals. Reading food labels and avoiding products with long lists of artificial ingredients can help reduce exposure to these inflammatory additives.

Highly Processed Foods: Highly processed foods, including fast food, frozen meals, convenience foods, and packaged snacks, often contain a combination of inflammatory ingredients such as refined grains, sugars, trans fats, and artificial additives. Choosing whole, minimally processed foods whenever possible can help reduce inflammation and promote overall health.

Allergens and Food Sensitivities: For individuals with food allergies or sensitivities, consuming certain foods can trigger an inflammatory response in the body. Common allergens include gluten, dairy, soy, eggs, peanuts, tree nuts, and shellfish. Identifying and avoiding trigger foods can help manage inflammation and reduce symptoms.

By becoming familiar with these common inflammatory foods and ingredients, individuals can make informed choices about their diet and prioritize foods that help reduce inflammation and support overall health and wellbeing.

Common inflammatory foods to avoid

Common inflammatory foods to avoid in order to reduce inflammation in the body include:

Refined Carbohydrates: Foods made with refined grains and sugars, such as white bread, white rice, pasta, sugary snacks, pastries, and desserts. These foods have a high glycemic index and can lead to spikes in blood sugar levels, promoting inflammation and insulin resistance.

Processed Meats: Processed meats such as bacon, sausage, hot dogs, deli meats, and canned meats. These meats often contain additives, preservatives, and high levels of saturated fats and sodium, which can promote inflammation and increase the risk of chronic diseases.

Trans Fats: Trans fats, also known as partially hydrogenated oils, are commonly found in fried foods, packaged snacks, margarine, shortening, and baked goods. These fats are highly inflammatory and have been linked to increased inflammation, insulin resistance, and cardiovascular disease risk.

Saturated Fats: While some sources of saturated fats may have neutral or even anti-inflammatory effects, excessive consumption of saturated fats from sources such as red meat, full-fat dairy, butter, and cheese can promote inflammation and increase the risk of chronic diseases.

Omega-6 Fatty Acids: Omega-6 fatty acids, found in vegetable oils such as soybean oil, corn oil, and sunflower oil, are essential fats that should be consumed in moderation. However, an imbalance between omega-6 and omega-3 fatty acids in the diet can promote inflammation. Limiting intake of omega-6-rich oils and focusing on increasing intake of omega-3 fatty acids from sources such as fatty fish, flaxseeds, and walnuts can help reduce inflammation.

Artificial Additives and Preservatives: Many processed and packaged foods contain artificial additives, preservatives, flavorings, and colorings that can trigger inflammation in sensitive individuals. Reading food labels and avoiding products with long lists of artificial ingredients can help reduce exposure to these inflammatory additives.

Highly Processed Foods: Highly processed foods, including fast food, frozen meals, convenience foods, and packaged snacks, often contain a combination of inflammatory ingredients such as refined grains, sugars, trans fats, and artificial additives. Choosing whole, minimally processed foods whenever possible can help reduce inflammation and promote overall health.

Allergens and Food Sensitivities: For individuals with food allergies or sensitivities, consuming certain foods can trigger an inflammatory response in the body. Common allergens include gluten, dairy, soy, eggs, peanuts, tree nuts, and shellfish. Identifying and avoiding trigger foods can help manage inflammation and reduce symptoms.

By avoiding these common inflammatory foods and ingredients, individuals can help reduce inflammation in the body and support overall health and wellbeing.

Reading food labels for hidden inflammatory ingredients

Reading food labels is essential for identifying hidden inflammatory ingredients and making informed choices about the foods we consume. Here are some tips for reading food labels to avoid inflammatory ingredients:

Check the Ingredient List: The ingredient list on food labels provides valuable information about the contents of the product. Look for common inflammatory ingredients such as refined grains, sugars, trans fats, artificial additives, and preservatives. Ingredients are listed in descending order by weight, so the first few ingredients make up the majority of the product.

Watch Out for Hidden Sugars: Sugar can hide under many different names on food labels, including sucrose, high-fructose corn syrup, cane sugar, maltose, dextrose, and fruit juice concentrate. Be vigilant in checking for these hidden sugars, especially in processed foods, sauces, dressings, and beverages.

Avoid Trans Fats: Trans fats are often listed on food labels as partially hydrogenated oils. Check the ingredient list for any mention of partially hydrogenated oils, as these fats are highly inflammatory and should be avoided.

Limit Saturated Fats: While some saturated fats are naturally present in foods like dairy and meat, excessive intake of saturated fats can promote inflammation. Check the saturated fat content on the nutrition label and opt for products with lower saturated fat content whenever possible.

Look for Whole, Minimally Processed Ingredients: Choose foods with simple, whole food ingredients and minimal processing. Ingredients you recognize and can pronounce are typically healthier choices than highly processed ingredients with long chemical names.

Beware of Artificial Additives and Preservatives: Scan the ingredient list for artificial additives, preservatives, flavorings, and colorings. Ingredients such as monosodium glutamate (MSG), artificial sweeteners, and food dyes have been linked to inflammation and other health issues.

Consider Allergens and Sensitivities: If you have food allergies or sensitivities, carefully check food labels for potential allergens such as gluten, dairy, soy, eggs, nuts, and shellfish. Food labels are required to clearly indicate the presence of common allergens to help consumers make safe choices.

Review Nutrition Facts: In addition to the ingredient list, review the nutrition facts panel for information on key nutrients such as sugar, fat, sodium, fiber, and protein. Pay attention to serving sizes and avoid products with excessive amounts of added sugars, saturated fats, and sodium.

By reading food labels carefully and being mindful of hidden inflammatory ingredients, you can make healthier choices that support inflammation reduction and overall wellbeing.

How cooking methods affect inflammation in foods

Methods

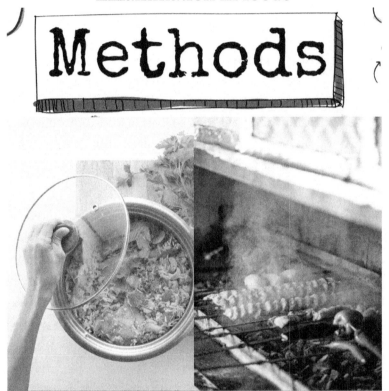

Cooking methods can influence the inflammatory properties of foods by altering their nutrient content, chemical composition, and formation of potentially harmful compounds. Here's how different cooking methods can impact inflammation in foods:

High-Heat Cooking: Cooking methods that involve high temperatures, such as frying, grilling, broiling, and barbecuing, can lead to the formation of advanced glycation end products (AGEs) and heterocyclic amines (HCAs). AGEs and HCAs are compounds that have been linked to inflammation and oxidative stress in the body. Limiting consumption of foods cooked at high temperatures can help reduce exposure to these inflammatory compounds.

Boiling and Steaming: Boiling and steaming are gentler cooking methods that involve cooking foods in water or steam at lower temperatures. These methods help preserve the nutrient content of foods and minimize the formation of AGEs and HCAs. Boiling and steaming are particularly suitable for vegetables, fish, and legumes, as they retain their texture, flavor, and nutritional value.

Sautéing and Stir-Frying: Sautéing and stir-frying involve cooking foods in a small amount of oil over medium to high heat. While these methods can help enhance the flavor and texture of foods, excessive heating of oils can lead to the formation of oxidized fats and free radicals, which can promote inflammation and oxidative stress. Using stable cooking oils with high smoke points, such as olive oil or avocado oil, and minimizing cooking time can help reduce the formation of harmful compounds.

Microwaving: Microwaving is a quick and convenient cooking method that involves using electromagnetic waves to heat food. While microwaving is generally considered safe and preserves the nutrient content of foods well, it may not be suitable for all types of foods or cooking tasks. Some studies suggest that microwaving may cause minor nutrient loss, but it is unlikely to significantly impact the inflammatory properties of foods.

Baking and Roasting: Baking and roasting foods in the oven at moderate temperatures can help retain their flavor, texture, and nutritional value. However, prolonged cooking times or high temperatures can lead to the formation of AGEs and HCAs, especially in meats and starchy foods. Using lower temperatures and shorter cooking times, marinating meats, and incorporating antioxidant-rich ingredients such as herbs, spices, and citrus can help mitigate the formation of harmful compounds.

Raw Foods: Eating raw or minimally processed foods can help preserve their natural enzymes, vitamins, minerals, and phytonutrients. However, some raw foods may be harder to digest or contain naturally occurring toxins or anti-nutrients that can trigger inflammation in sensitive individuals. Cooking certain foods can help break down these compounds and enhance their nutritional value.

Overall, choosing cooking methods that involve lower temperatures, shorter cooking times, and minimal exposure to harmful compounds can help reduce inflammation in foods and promote overall health and wellbeing. Additionally, incorporating a variety of fruits, vegetables, whole grains, lean proteins, and healthy fats into your diet can provide a diverse array of nutrients and antioxidants to support inflammation reduction.

STOCKING YOUR PANTRY AND KITCHEN FOR SUCCESS

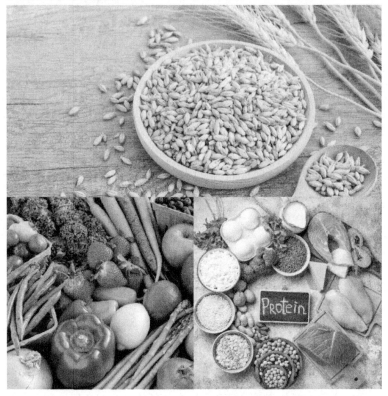

Stocking your pantry and kitchen with the right ingredients can set you up for success when following an anti-inflammatory diet. Here's a guide to stocking your pantry and kitchen for inflammation reduction:

1. Whole Grains:

Brown rice

Quinoa

Oats

Barley

Whole wheat pasta

Buckwheat

Bulgur

Millet

2. Healthy Fats:

Extra virgin olive oil

Avocado oil

Coconut oil (in moderation)

Nuts (almonds, walnuts, pistachios)

Seeds (flaxseeds, chia seeds, hemp seeds)

Nut butters (almond butter, peanut butter)

3. Lean Proteins:

Skinless poultry (chicken, turkey)

Fish (salmon, mackerel, sardines, trout)

Tofu

Tempeh

Legumes (beans, lentils, chickpeas)

Eggs

4. Fruits and Vegetables:

Fresh fruits (berries, apples, oranges, bananas)

Leafy greens (spinach, kale, arugula)

Cruciferous vegetables (broccoli, cauliflower, Brussels sprouts)

Colorful vegetables (bell peppers, tomatoes, carrots)

Berries (blueberries, strawberries, raspberries)

Citrus fruits (lemons, limes, oranges)

5. Herbs and Spices:

Turmeric

Ginger

Garlic

Cinnamon

Rosemary

Basil

Oregano

Thyme

6. Whole Food Condiments:

Balsamic vinegar

Apple cider vinegar

Dijon mustard

Tamari or soy sauce (choose low-sodium options)

Tomato paste

Salsa (without added sugar)

7. Non-Dairy Milk Alternatives:

Almond milk

Coconut milk

Soy milk (choose unsweetened varieties)

Oat milk

8. Whole Grains and Legumes:

Whole wheat flour

Whole grain bread and wraps

Rolled oats

Lentils

Beans (black beans, kidney beans, chickpeas)

Quinoa

9. Canned and Jarred Goods:

Canned beans (rinse well to reduce sodium)

Canned tomatoes

Jarred olives

Jarred roasted red peppers

Unsweetened applesauce

10. Healthy Snacks:

Raw nuts and seeds

Fresh fruit

Veggie sticks with hummus

Air-popped popcorn

Whole grain crackers

Dark chocolate (70% or higher cocoa content)

11. Cooking Essentials:

Low-sodium vegetable or chicken broth

Dried herbs and spices

Sea salt or Himalayan pink salt

Black pepper

Baking staples (baking powder, baking soda, vanilla extract)

By stocking your pantry and kitchen with these anti-inflammatory ingredients, you'll have a wide range of options for creating nutritious and delicious meals that support inflammation reduction and overall health and wellbeing. Remember to prioritize whole, minimally processed foods and choose organic options whenever possible to minimize exposure to pesticides and other potentially harmful substances.

Essential pantry staples for an anti-inflammatory diet

For an anti-inflammatory diet, it's essential to stock your pantry with nutrient-dense, whole foods that help reduce inflammation and promote overall health. Here are some essential pantry staples for an anti-inflammatory diet:

Whole Grains:

Brown rice

Quinoa

Oats

Barley

Whole wheat pasta

Buckwheat

Bulgur

Millet

Healthy Fats:

Extra virgin olive oil

Avocado oil

Coconut oil (in moderation)

Nuts (almonds, walnuts, pistachios)

Seeds (flaxseeds, chia seeds, hemp seeds)

Nut butters (almond butter, peanut butter)

Lean Proteins:

Skinless poultry (chicken, turkey)

Fish (salmon, mackerel, sardines, trout)

Tofu

Tempeh

Legumes (beans, lentils, chickpeas)

Eggs

Fruits and Vegetables:

Fresh fruits (berries, apples, oranges, bananas)

Leafy greens (spinach, kale, arugula)

Cruciferous vegetables (broccoli, cauliflower, Brussels sprouts)

Colorful vegetables (bell peppers, tomatoes, carrots)

Berries (blueberries, strawberries, raspberries)

Citrus fruits (lemons, limes, oranges)

Herbs and Spices:

Turmeric

Ginger

Garlic

Cinnamon

Rosemary

Basil

Oregano

Thyme

Whole Food Condiments:

Balsamic vinegar

Apple cider vinegar

Dijon mustard

Tamari or soy sauce (choose low-sodium options)

Tomato paste

Salsa (without added sugar)

Non-Dairy Milk Alternatives:

Almond milk

Coconut milk

Soy milk (choose unsweetened varieties)

Oat milk

Whole Grains and Legumes:

Whole wheat flour

Whole grain bread and wraps

Rolled oats

Lentils

Beans (black beans, kidney beans, chickpeas)

Quinoa

Canned and Jarred Goods:

Canned beans (rinse well to reduce sodium)

Canned tomatoes

Jarred olives

Jarred roasted red peppers

Unsweetened applesauce

Healthy Snacks:

Raw nuts and seeds

Fresh fruit

Veggie sticks with hummus

Air-popped popcorn

Whole grain crackers

Dark chocolate (70% or higher cocoa content)

Cooking Essentials:

Low-sodium vegetable or chicken broth

Dried herbs and spices

Sea salt or Himalayan pink salt

Black pepper

Baking staples (baking powder, baking soda, vanilla extract)

By keeping these essential pantry staples on hand, you'll have a variety of ingredients to create nutritious and flavorful meals that support inflammation reduction and promote overall health and wellbeing. Remember to prioritize whole, minimally processed foods and choose organic options whenever possible to maximize nutritional benefits.

Tools and kitchen equipment for meal preparation

Having the right tools and kitchen equipment can make meal preparation more efficient and enjoyable. Here are some essential tools and equipment for cooking healthy, anti-inflammatory meals:

Chef's Knife: A high-quality chef's knife is essential for chopping, slicing, and dicing fruits, vegetables, and proteins.

Cutting Board: Choose a sturdy cutting board made of wood, bamboo, or plastic for chopping ingredients safely.

Vegetable Peeler: A vegetable peeler makes it easy to peel and prep fruits and vegetables.

Mixing Bowls: Stainless steel or glass mixing bowls in various sizes are useful for mixing, marinating, and storing ingredients.

Measuring Cups and Spoons: Accurate measuring cups and spoons are essential for portion control and following recipes.

Whisk: A whisk is handy for blending ingredients, emulsifying dressings, and whipping eggs.

Spatula: A heat-resistant spatula is essential for flipping, stirring, and scraping ingredients in pans and pots.

Non-Stick Skillet or Pan: A non-stick skillet or pan makes cooking with less oil possible and is ideal for sautéing vegetables and cooking proteins.

Baking Sheet: A sturdy baking sheet is essential for roasting vegetables, baking proteins, and making one-pan meals.

Pot and Saucepan Set: A set of pots and saucepans in various sizes is essential for cooking grains, boiling vegetables, and making soups and sauces.

Steamer Basket: A steamer basket is useful for steaming vegetables while preserving their nutrients and texture.

Blender or Food Processor: A blender or food processor is versatile for making smoothies, sauces, soups, dips, and nut butters.

Immersion Blender: An immersion blender is handy for blending soups, sauces, and smoothies directly in the pot or container.

Slow Cooker or Instant Pot: A slow cooker or Instant Pot is convenient for cooking flavorful and tender meals with minimal effort.

Grater or Microplane: A grater or microplane is useful for grating cheese, zesting citrus fruits, and shredding vegetables.

Salad Spinner: A salad spinner makes washing and drying leafy greens quick and easy.

Oven Thermometer: An oven thermometer ensures accurate oven temperature for baking and roasting.

Kitchen Timer: A kitchen timer helps you keep track of cooking times and prevents overcooking.

Tongs: Tongs are versatile for flipping, turning, and serving foods, especially on the grill or stovetop.

Silicone Baking Mats: Silicone baking mats provide a non-stick surface for baking and roasting without the need for parchment paper or cooking spray.

With these essential tools and kitchen equipment, you'll be well-equipped to prepare delicious and nutritious meals that support inflammation reduction and promote overall health and wellbeing.

Tips for grocery shopping and meal planning

Here are some tips for effective grocery shopping and meal planning to support your anti-inflammatory diet:

Plan Ahead: Take some time to plan your meals for the week before heading to the grocery store. Consider your schedule, dietary preferences, and any special occasions or events.

Make a Shopping List: Create a detailed shopping list based on your meal plan and the ingredients you need. Organize your list by categories such as produce, pantry staples, proteins, dairy, and frozen foods to make shopping more efficient.

Focus on Whole Foods: Prioritize whole, minimally processed foods such as fruits, vegetables, whole grains, lean proteins, nuts, seeds, and healthy fats. Choose organic options whenever possible to minimize exposure to pesticides and other potentially harmful substances.

Read Food Labels: When selecting packaged and processed foods, read food labels carefully to avoid products with added sugars, unhealthy fats, artificial additives, and preservatives. Look for products with simple, recognizable ingredients and minimal processing.

Shop the Perimeter: In most grocery stores, the perimeter is where you'll find fresh produce, meats, dairy, and other whole foods. Spend the majority of your time shopping in this area to stock up on nutrient-dense ingredients.

Include a Variety of Colors: Aim to include a variety of colorful fruits and vegetables in your shopping cart to ensure a diverse array of nutrients and antioxidants. Choose a rainbow of colors, including greens, reds, oranges, yellows, blues, and purples.

Buy in Bulk: Consider purchasing staple items such as grains, legumes, nuts, and seeds in bulk to save money and reduce packaging waste. Store bulk items in airtight containers to maintain freshness.

Stock Up on Frozen Produce: Frozen fruits and vegetables are convenient, budget-friendly, and often just as nutritious as fresh produce. Stock up on frozen options to have on hand for quick and easy meal preparation.

Choose Healthy Snacks: Opt for nutrient-dense snacks such as fresh fruit, raw nuts and seeds, veggie sticks with hummus, Greek yogurt, and whole grain crackers. Avoid highly processed snacks with added sugars, unhealthy fats, and artificial ingredients.

Meal Prep in Advance: Set aside time each week to prepare and portion out ingredients for meals and snacks. Wash, chop, and store fruits and vegetables, cook grains and proteins, and assemble grab-and-go snacks to streamline meal preparation throughout the week.

Be Flexible: While it's important to plan ahead, be flexible and open to making adjustments based on seasonal availability, sales, and your individual preferences. Don't be afraid to experiment with new recipes and ingredients to keep meals exciting and enjoyable.

By following these tips, you can make grocery shopping and meal planning easier, more efficient, and more enjoyable while supporting your anti-inflammatory diet goals.

BUILDING BALANCED MEALS: RECIPES AND MEAL PLANS

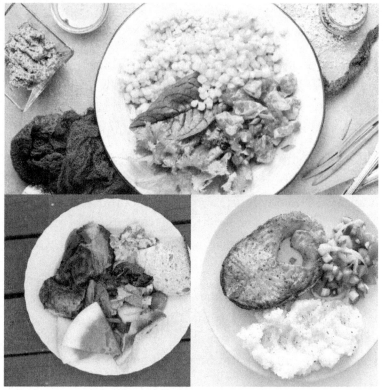

Building balanced meals is key to supporting an anti-inflammatory diet and promoting overall health and wellbeing. Here are some recipe ideas and sample meal plans to help you create balanced meals that incorporate anti-inflammatory ingredients:

Recipe Ideas:

Grilled Salmon with Quinoa and Roasted Vegetables:

Grilled salmon seasoned with lemon, garlic, and herbs

Quinoa cooked with low-sodium vegetable broth

Roasted mixed vegetables (such as bell peppers, zucchini, and carrots) tossed with olive oil and herbs

Vegetable Stir-Fry with Tofu:

Tofu stir-fried with mixed vegetables (such as broccoli, bell peppers, snap peas, and mushrooms)

Brown rice or quinoa as a base

Stir-fry sauce made with low-sodium soy sauce, ginger, garlic, and sesame oil

Mediterranean Chickpea Salad:

Mixed greens topped with chickpeas, cherry tomatoes, cucumber, red onion, and Kalamata olives

Crumbled feta cheese

Lemon-tahini dressing made with lemon juice, tahini, garlic, and olive oil

Turkey and Vegetable Chili:

Ground turkey cooked with onions, bell peppers, tomatoes, beans, and spices (such as chili powder, cumin, and paprika)

Serve with a dollop of Greek yogurt or avocado slices for creaminess

Whole grain cornbread on the side

Quinoa and Black Bean Stuffed Bell Peppers:

Bell peppers stuffed with cooked quinoa, black beans, corn, diced tomatoes, and spices

Baked until tender and topped with fresh cilantro and a squeeze of lime juice

Serve with a side of mixed greens or a green salad

Sample Meal Plans:

Day 1:

Breakfast: Greek yogurt topped with fresh berries, sliced almonds, and a drizzle of honey

Lunch: Mediterranean Chickpea Salad with lemon-tahini dressing

Dinner: Grilled Salmon with Quinoa and Roasted Vegetables

Day 2:

Breakfast: Green smoothie made with spinach, kale, banana, almond milk, and chia seeds

Lunch: Turkey and Vegetable Chili with a side of whole grain cornbread

Dinner: Vegetable Stir-Fry with Tofu served over brown rice

Day 3:

Breakfast: Oatmeal topped with sliced banana, walnuts, and a sprinkle of cinnamon

Lunch: Quinoa and Black Bean Stuffed Bell Peppers with a side of mixed greens

Dinner: Baked chicken breast seasoned with herbs, roasted sweet potatoes, and steamed broccoli

Day 4:

Breakfast: Scrambled eggs with sautéed spinach, tomatoes, and mushrooms

Lunch: Lentil and Vegetable Soup with whole grain bread

Dinner: Whole wheat pasta with marinara sauce, grilled chicken breast, and a side salad

By incorporating a variety of nutrient-dense ingredients and balanced meals into your diet, you can support inflammation reduction and promote optimal health and wellbeing.

Breakfast recipes and meal ideas

Here are some delicious and nutritious breakfast recipes and meal ideas that incorporate anti-inflammatory ingredients:

Green Smoothie Bowl:

Blend together spinach, kale, banana, frozen berries, almond milk, and a scoop of protein powder until smooth.

Pour into a bowl and top with sliced fresh fruit, granola, shredded coconut, and a sprinkle of chia seeds.

Turmeric Oatmeal:

Cook rolled oats with water or almond milk until creamy.

Stir in ground turmeric, cinnamon, ginger, and a pinch of black pepper for enhanced absorption.

Top with sliced almonds, chopped dates, and a drizzle of honey or maple syrup.

Avocado Toast with Poached Egg:

Toast whole grain bread and top with mashed avocado, a squeeze of lemon juice, and a sprinkle of red pepper flakes.

Poach an egg and place it on top of the avocado toast.

Garnish with chopped fresh herbs, such as cilantro or parsley, and a sprinkle of sea salt and black pepper.

Berry Chia Seed Pudding:

Mix together chia seeds, almond milk, vanilla extract, and a touch of honey or maple syrup in a jar or bowl.

Stir in a handful of mixed berries (such as strawberries, blueberries, and raspberries).

Let the mixture sit in the refrigerator overnight to thicken.

Serve the next morning topped with additional berries and a dollop of Greek yogurt, if desired.

Smoked Salmon Breakfast Wrap:

Spread hummus or mashed avocado on a whole grain wrap or tortilla.

Layer with smoked salmon, sliced cucumber, tomato, red onion, and baby spinach.

Roll up the wrap and enjoy as a satisfying and protein-rich breakfast.

Coconut Yogurt Parfait:

Layer coconut yogurt with fresh mango chunks, toasted coconut flakes, and a sprinkle of chopped nuts or seeds in a glass or jar.

Repeat the layers until the jar is filled.

Drizzle with honey or maple syrup for added sweetness, if desired.

Quinoa Breakfast Bowl:

Cook quinoa with coconut milk and a dash of cinnamon until fluffy.

Top with sliced bananas, toasted almonds, shredded coconut, and a drizzle of almond butter or tahini.

Optional: Stir in a spoonful of Greek yogurt for creaminess.

Sweet Potato Breakfast Hash:

Sauté diced sweet potatoes with bell peppers, onions, and spinach in olive oil until tender.

Season with smoked paprika, garlic powder, and cumin.

Serve topped with a fried or poached egg and a sprinkle of fresh herbs.

These breakfast recipes and meal ideas are not only delicious but also packed with nutrients and anti-inflammatory ingredients to help you start your day on the right foot. Feel free to customize them based on your preferences and dietary needs.

Lunch recipes and meal ideas

Here are some flavorful and nutritious lunch recipes and meal ideas featuring anti-inflammatory ingredients:

Mediterranean Quinoa Salad:

Cook quinoa according to package instructions and let it cool.

Mix the cooked quinoa with chopped cucumber, cherry tomatoes, Kalamata olives, red onion, and crumbled feta cheese.

Dress with a lemon-olive oil vinaigrette and garnish with fresh parsley and a sprinkle of dried oregano.

Grilled Chicken and Veggie Wrap:

Grill or roast chicken breast seasoned with lemon, garlic, and herbs until cooked through.

Spread hummus or Greek yogurt on a whole grain wrap or tortilla.

Layer with sliced grilled chicken, roasted vegetables (such as bell peppers, zucchini, and eggplant), and baby spinach.

Roll up the wrap and slice in half for a satisfying and portable lunch.

Rainbow Buddha Bowl:

Fill a bowl with cooked quinoa or brown rice as the base.

Top with a variety of colorful vegetables (such as roasted sweet potatoes, steamed broccoli, shredded carrots, and raw bell peppers).

Add a serving of protein (such as grilled tofu, chickpeas, or edamame).

Drizzle with tahini or avocado dressing and sprinkle with sesame seeds or chopped nuts for crunch.

Salmon Salad with Avocado Dressing:

Grill or bake salmon fillets seasoned with lemon, garlic, and dill until flaky.

Toss mixed greens with sliced cucumber, cherry tomatoes, avocado chunks, and thinly sliced red onion.

Top the salad with the cooked salmon and drizzle with a creamy avocado dressing made with avocado, Greek yogurt, lime juice, and cilantro.

Vegetarian Lentil Soup:

Sauté diced onions, carrots, and celery in olive oil until softened.

Add dried green or brown lentils, low-sodium vegetable broth, diced tomatoes, and your favorite herbs and spices (such as thyme, rosemary, and bay leaves).

Simmer until the lentils are tender and the flavors are well combined.

Serve hot with a slice of whole grain bread or a side of mixed greens.

Asian-Inspired Tofu Stir-Fry:

Press tofu to remove excess moisture and cut into cubes.

Stir-fry tofu with mixed vegetables (such as bell peppers, snap peas, broccoli, and carrots) in a wok or skillet.

Season with a sauce made from low-sodium soy sauce, rice vinegar, garlic, ginger, and a touch of honey or maple syrup.

Serve over cooked brown rice or quinoa and garnish with sliced green onions and sesame seeds.

Greek Chickpea Salad Sandwich:

Mash cooked chickpeas with Greek yogurt, lemon juice, chopped cucumber, red onion, and fresh dill.

Spread the chickpea salad on whole grain bread and top with sliced tomatoes, lettuce, and cucumber slices.

Serve as a hearty and protein-packed sandwich for lunch.

These lunch recipes and meal ideas are both satisfying and nutritious, providing a balance of protein, fiber, healthy fats, and essential nutrients to keep you energized throughout the day. Feel free to customize them based on your preferences and dietary needs.

Dinner recipes and meal ideas

Here are some delicious and satisfying dinner recipes and meal ideas featuring anti-inflammatory ingredients:

Baked Salmon with Roasted Vegetables:

Season salmon fillets with olive oil, lemon juice, garlic, and dill.

Bake in the oven until the salmon is cooked through and flakes easily with a fork.

Serve with a side of roasted vegetables, such as broccoli, cauliflower, and carrots, tossed with olive oil, garlic, and herbs.

Vegetable and Chickpea Curry:

Sauté diced onions, bell peppers, and carrots in coconut oil until softened.

Add curry powder, turmeric, cumin, ginger, and garlic and cook until fragrant.

Stir in diced tomatoes, coconut milk, and cooked chickpeas.

Simmer until the flavors are well combined and the sauce has thickened.

Serve over cooked brown rice or quinoa and garnish with fresh cilantro.

Grilled Chicken with Greek Salad:

Marinate chicken breast in olive oil, lemon juice, oregano, garlic, and black pepper.

Grill until cooked through and lightly charred on the outside.

Serve with a refreshing Greek salad made with mixed greens, cherry tomatoes, cucumber, red onion, Kalamata olives, and feta cheese.

Drizzle with a simple vinaigrette made from olive oil, red wine vinegar, Dijon mustard, and dried oregano.

Stuffed Bell Peppers with Quinoa and Black Beans:

Cook quinoa according to package instructions and set aside.

Cut the tops off bell peppers and remove the seeds and membranes.

In a bowl, mix cooked quinoa with black beans, corn, diced tomatoes, chopped cilantro, and Mexican spices (such as chili powder, cumin, and paprika).

Stuff the bell peppers with the quinoa mixture and bake in the oven until the peppers are tender.

Serve with a dollop of Greek yogurt or avocado slices on top.

Eggplant and Chickpea Tagine:

Sauté diced onions, garlic, and ginger in olive oil until softened.

Add diced eggplant, chickpeas, diced tomatoes, vegetable broth, and Moroccan spices (such as cumin, coriander, cinnamon, and paprika).

Simmer until the eggplant is tender and the flavors have melded together.

Serve over cooked couscous or quinoa and garnish with chopped fresh parsley and a squeeze of lemon juice.

Tofu and Vegetable Stir-Fry with Peanut Sauce:

Stir-fry tofu cubes with mixed vegetables (such as bell peppers, broccoli, snap peas, and carrots) in a wok or skillet.

Make a simple peanut sauce by whisking together peanut butter, soy sauce, lime juice, garlic, ginger, and a touch of honey or maple syrup.

Toss the stir-fried tofu and vegetables with the peanut sauce until well coated.

Serve over cooked brown rice or noodles and garnish with chopped peanuts and green onions.

Mediterranean Turkey Meatballs with Tzatziki Sauce:

Mix ground turkey with minced garlic, chopped parsley, oregano, lemon zest, and breadcrumbs.

Form into meatballs and bake in the oven until cooked through.

Serve with homemade tzatziki sauce made from Greek yogurt, grated cucumber, lemon juice, dill, and garlic.

Enjoy with a side of whole wheat pita bread and a Greek salad.

These dinner recipes and meal ideas are nutritious, flavorful, and easy to prepare, making them perfect for busy weeknights or relaxed weekends. Feel free to customize them based on your preferences and dietary needs.

Snack options for an anti-inflammatory diet

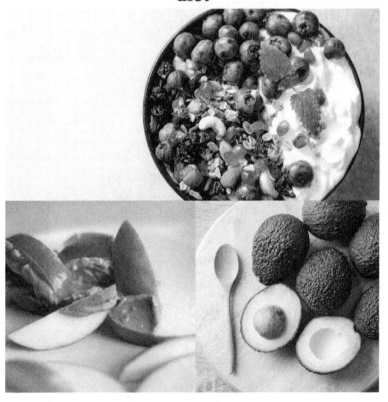

Here are some healthy and satisfying snack options that are perfect for an anti-inflammatory diet:

Raw Vegetables with Hummus:

Serve sliced bell peppers, cucumber, carrots, and cherry tomatoes with a side of hummus for dipping. Hummus is made from chickpeas, which are rich in fiber and anti-inflammatory nutrients.

Greek Yogurt with Berries and Almonds:

Enjoy a serving of Greek yogurt topped with fresh berries (such as strawberries, blueberries, or raspberries) and a sprinkle of almonds. Greek yogurt is high in protein and probiotics, while berries are packed with antioxidants.

Apple Slices with Almond Butter:

Spread almond butter on apple slices for a crunchy and satisfying snack. Almonds are rich in healthy fats and vitamin E, which have anti-inflammatory properties, while apples provide fiber and vitamins.

Avocado Toast:

Spread mashed avocado on whole grain toast and sprinkle with sea salt and red pepper flakes. Avocado is loaded with monounsaturated fats and potassium, which can help reduce inflammation.

Trail Mix:

Mix together a combination of raw nuts (such as almonds, walnuts, and cashews), seeds (such as pumpkin seeds and sunflower seeds), and dried fruits (such as raisins, apricots, and cranberries) for a portable and nutritious snack.

Chia Seed Pudding:

Make chia seed pudding by mixing chia seeds with almond milk, vanilla extract, and a touch of honey or maple syrup. Let it sit in the refrigerator until thickened, then top with fresh fruit and a sprinkle of cinnamon.

Edamame:

Enjoy steamed edamame pods sprinkled with sea salt for a protein-rich snack. Edamame is a good source of plant-based protein and isoflavones, which have anti-inflammatory effects.

Roasted Chickpeas:

Toss cooked chickpeas with olive oil and spices (such as cumin, paprika, and garlic powder) and roast in the oven until crispy. Chickpeas are high in fiber and protein and can help lower markers of inflammation in the body.

Dark Chocolate:

Indulge in a square or two of dark chocolate (70% or higher cocoa content) for a sweet treat. Dark chocolate is rich in flavonoids, which have antioxidant and anti-inflammatory properties.

Seaweed Snacks:

Enjoy crispy seaweed snacks seasoned with sea salt or sesame oil for a savory and nutritious snack. Seaweed is packed with vitamins, minerals, and antioxidants that can help reduce inflammation.

These snack options are not only delicious but also packed with nutrients and anti-inflammatory ingredients to help keep you satisfied between meals. Incorporate a variety of these snacks into your daily routine to support your anti-inflammatory diet goals.

INCORPORATING ANTI-INFLAMMATORY FOODS INTO YOUR DIET

Incorporating anti-inflammatory foods into your diet is a great way to support overall health and wellbeing. Here are some tips to help you add more anti-inflammatory foods to your meals:

Focus on Whole Foods: Choose whole, minimally processed foods such as fruits, vegetables, whole grains, lean proteins, nuts, seeds, and healthy fats. These foods are rich in vitamins, minerals, antioxidants, and phytochemicals that can help reduce inflammation in the body.

Eat Plenty of Fruits and Vegetables: Aim to fill half of your plate with colorful fruits and vegetables at each meal. Choose a variety of colors to ensure you're getting a wide range of nutrients and antioxidants. Berries, leafy greens, cruciferous vegetables, and citrus fruits are particularly high in anti-inflammatory compounds.

Include Omega-3 Fatty Acids: Incorporate sources of omega-3 fatty acids into your diet, such as fatty fish (salmon, mackerel, sardines), walnuts, flaxseeds, chia seeds, and hemp seeds. Omega-3 fatty acids have been shown to have anti-inflammatory effects and may help reduce the risk of chronic diseases.

Add Herbs and Spices: Use herbs and spices liberally in your cooking to add flavor and anti-inflammatory benefits to your meals. Turmeric, ginger, garlic, cinnamon, cumin, and rosemary are particularly potent anti-inflammatory spices that can be easily incorporated into a variety of dishes.

Choose Healthy Fats: Opt for sources of healthy fats such as olive oil, avocado, nuts, and seeds. These fats are rich in monounsaturated and polyunsaturated fats, which have been shown to have anti-inflammatory effects and may help lower levels of inflammation in the body.

Limit Added Sugars and Refined Carbohydrates: Reduce your intake of added sugars and refined carbohydrates, which can promote inflammation in the body. Instead, focus on whole, unprocessed carbohydrates such as whole grains, fruits, and vegetables, which provide fiber and nutrients without causing spikes in blood sugar levels.

Include Fermented Foods: Incorporate fermented foods such as yogurt, kefir, sauerkraut, kimchi, and miso into your diet. These foods contain beneficial probiotics that support gut health and may help reduce inflammation in the body.

Drink Green Tea: Enjoy green tea regularly as a beverage choice. Green tea is rich in antioxidants called catechins, which have anti-inflammatory and anti-cancer properties. Drinking green tea may help reduce inflammation and protect against chronic diseases.

Stay Hydrated: Drink plenty of water throughout the day to stay hydrated and support overall health. Adequate hydration is important for maintaining healthy bodily functions and may help reduce inflammation in the body.

Experiment with New Recipes: Be adventurous in the kitchen and try out new recipes that feature anti-inflammatory ingredients. Explore different cuisines and cooking methods to keep your meals exciting and flavorful while reaping the benefits of anti-inflammatory foods.

By incorporating these tips into your daily eating habits, you can create a balanced and nutritious diet that supports inflammation reduction and promotes optimal health and wellbeing. Remember to listen to your body and make choices that align with your individual preferences and dietary needs.

Top anti-inflammatory foods to include in your meals

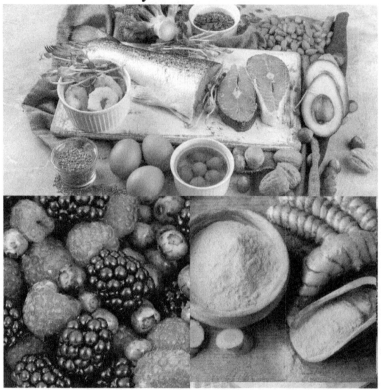

Here are some of the top anti-inflammatory foods that you can include in your meals to promote overall health and wellbeing:

Fatty Fish: Fatty fish such as salmon, mackerel, sardines, and trout are rich in omega-3 fatty acids, which have potent anti-inflammatory effects. Aim to include fatty fish in your diet at least two to three times per week.

Leafy Greens: Leafy green vegetables like spinach, kale, Swiss chard, and collard greens are packed with vitamins, minerals, and antioxidants that help combat inflammation. Add leafy greens to salads, smoothies, soups, and stir-fries for a nutritious boost.

Berries: Berries such as blueberries, strawberries, raspberries, and blackberries are loaded with antioxidants called anthocyanins, which have anti-inflammatory properties. Enjoy fresh berries as a snack, add them to yogurt or oatmeal, or blend them into smoothies.

Turmeric: Turmeric is a spice that contains curcumin, a compound known for its powerful anti-inflammatory and antioxidant properties. Add turmeric to curries, soups, stews, and smoothies to reap its health benefits.

Ginger: Ginger is another spice with potent anti-inflammatory properties. It contains compounds called gingerols, which have been shown to reduce inflammation and relieve pain. Use fresh ginger in stir-fries, teas, marinades, and dressings.

Nuts and Seeds: Nuts and seeds such as almonds, walnuts, flaxseeds, chia seeds, and hemp seeds are rich in healthy fats, fiber, and antioxidants that help reduce inflammation. Enjoy them as a snack, sprinkle them on salads or yogurt, or use them in homemade granola or energy bars.

Avocado: Avocado is a rich source of monounsaturated fats, which have anti-inflammatory effects. It also contains antioxidants and fiber that contribute to its anti-inflammatory properties. Add sliced avocado to salads, sandwiches, wraps, and smoothies.

Olive Oil: Extra virgin olive oil is rich in monounsaturated fats and contains compounds called polyphenols, which have anti-inflammatory and antioxidant effects. Use olive oil for cooking, salad dressings, and drizzling over roasted vegetables or whole grains.

Cruciferous Vegetables: Cruciferous vegetables such as broccoli, cauliflower, Brussels sprouts, and cabbage are rich in antioxidants and sulfur compounds that help reduce inflammation and detoxify the body. Incorporate them into stir-fries, salads, soups, and roasted vegetable dishes.

Tomatoes: Tomatoes are a great source of lycopene, a powerful antioxidant with anti-inflammatory properties. Enjoy tomatoes fresh in salads and sandwiches, cooked in sauces and soups, or roasted with olive oil and herbs.

Incorporating these top anti-inflammatory foods into your meals regularly can help support inflammation reduction, promote overall health, and reduce the risk of chronic diseases. Aim for a diverse and balanced diet that includes a variety of these nutrient-rich foods to maximize their health benefits.

Creative ways to incorporate more fruits and vegetables

Incorporating more fruits and vegetables into your diet can be both delicious and fun! Here are some creative ways to add more fruits and vegetables to your meals:

Smoothies and Smoothie Bowls: Blend together your favorite fruits and leafy greens with Greek yogurt, almond milk, or coconut water to create refreshing smoothies. You can also pour the smoothie into a bowl and top it with additional fruits, nuts, seeds, and granola for a satisfying smoothie bowl.

Zoodles: Use a spiralizer to turn zucchini, carrots, or sweet potatoes into noodles (zoodles). You can then use the zoodles as a nutritious alternative to traditional pasta in dishes like stir-fries, salads, and pasta sauces.

Stuffed Vegetables: Hollow out vegetables like bell peppers, tomatoes, zucchini, or mushrooms and stuff them with a mixture of grains, lean proteins, and herbs. Bake or grill until the vegetables are tender for a flavorful and nutritious meal.

Vegetable Chips: Slice vegetables like kale, sweet potatoes, beets, or carrots thinly, toss them with olive oil and your favorite seasonings, and bake until crispy. These homemade vegetable chips make a tasty and healthier alternative to store-bought potato chips.

Vegetable-Based Sauces and Dips: Use pureed vegetables like roasted red peppers, butternut squash, or cauliflower as a base for sauces and dips. Mix them with herbs, spices, and Greek yogurt or tahini for added flavor and creaminess.

Vegetable Wraps and Rolls: Use large lettuce leaves, collard greens, or nori sheets as wraps or rolls for filling with your favorite vegetables, proteins, and spreads. Roll them up tightly for a handheld, portable meal or snack.

Vegetable Pizza Crust: Make a pizza crust using cauliflower, sweet potatoes, or zucchini instead of traditional flour. Top the crust with tomato sauce, cheese, and plenty of colorful vegetables for a nutritious and satisfying pizza.

Stuffed Squash or Potatoes: Roast acorn squash, delicata squash, or sweet potatoes until tender, then fill them with a mixture of quinoa, beans, vegetables, and cheese. Bake until heated through for a hearty and comforting meal.

Fruit Salsas and Chutneys: Combine diced fruits like mango, pineapple, or peaches with onions, peppers, cilantro, and lime juice to make a vibrant salsa or chutney. Serve it as a topping for grilled meats, fish, tacos, or salads.

Vegetable Noodles in Soups: Add spiralized or thinly sliced vegetables like carrots, zucchini, or squash to soups and stews for added texture, color, and nutrients. They cook quickly and absorb the flavors of the broth, making them a tasty addition to any soup.

By getting creative in the kitchen and experimenting with different cooking techniques and recipes, you can easily incorporate more fruits and vegetables into your meals and enjoy the health benefits they provide.

Protein sources that reduce inflammation

Incorporating protein sources that help reduce inflammation can be beneficial for overall health and wellbeing. Here are some protein-rich foods that are known for their anti-inflammatory properties:

Fatty Fish: Salmon, mackerel, sardines, trout, and herring are rich in omega-3 fatty acids, which have been shown to reduce inflammation in the body. Aim to include fatty fish in your diet at least two to three times per week.

Legumes: Beans, lentils, chickpeas, and peas are excellent plant-based sources of protein that also contain fiber and phytonutrients with anti-inflammatory properties. They can help lower levels of inflammatory markers in the body when consumed regularly.

Tofu and Tempeh: Tofu and tempeh are soy-based protein sources that provide a complete source of protein along with beneficial phytonutrients called isoflavones. Soy products have been associated with reduced inflammation and may help protect against chronic diseases.

Nuts and Seeds: Almonds, walnuts, flaxseeds, chia seeds, hemp seeds, and pumpkin seeds are rich in protein, healthy fats, and antioxidants that have anti-inflammatory effects. They can be enjoyed as snacks, added to salads, or used in recipes to boost protein intake.

Quinoa: Quinoa is a gluten-free whole grain that is also a complete source of protein, meaning it contains all nine essential amino acids. It is rich in fiber, vitamins, and minerals, and has anti-inflammatory properties that can help reduce inflammation in the body.

Greek Yogurt: Greek yogurt is high in protein and probiotics, which promote gut health and may help reduce inflammation. Choose plain Greek yogurt without added sugars and flavor it with fresh fruit, nuts, or honey for a nutritious snack or breakfast option.

Eggs: Eggs are a versatile and affordable source of high-quality protein that also contain vitamins, minerals, and antioxidants. They can be enjoyed boiled, scrambled, poached, or added to salads and sandwiches for a protein boost.

Incorporating these protein sources into your diet regularly can help support inflammation reduction and promote overall health and wellbeing. Aim for a balanced diet that includes a variety of protein-rich foods along with plenty of fruits, vegetables, and whole grains for optimal health.

LIFESTYLE CHANGES FOR REDUCING INFLAMMATION

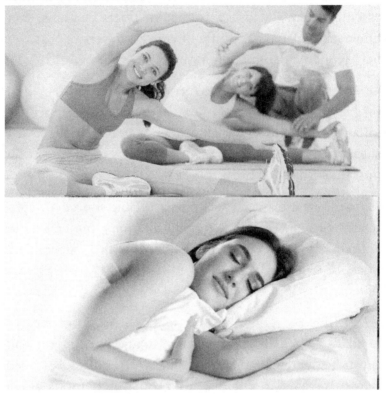

Making lifestyle changes to incorporate regular exercise, manage stress effectively, and prioritize quality sleep can all contribute to reducing inflammation in the body. Here's how each of these factors plays a role in inflammation reduction:

Regular Exercise:

Engaging in regular physical activity has been shown to have anti-inflammatory effects on the body. Exercise helps reduce inflammation by promoting circulation, improving insulin sensitivity, and modulating the immune response.

Aim for at least 150 minutes of moderate-intensity aerobic exercise or 75 minutes of vigorous-intensity aerobic exercise each week, along with muscle-strengthening activities on two or more days per week.

Choose activities you enjoy, such as walking, jogging, swimming, cycling, yoga, or strength training, and make exercise a regular part of your routine.

Stress Management:

Chronic stress can trigger inflammation in the body and contribute to the development of inflammatory conditions. Finding effective ways to manage stress can help reduce inflammation and promote overall wellbeing.

Practice stress-reduction techniques such as deep breathing exercises, meditation, mindfulness, progressive muscle relaxation, or yoga to calm the mind and body.

Engage in activities that you find relaxing and enjoyable, such as spending time in nature, listening to music, practicing hobbies, or spending quality time with loved ones.

Quality Sleep:

Getting enough high-quality sleep is essential for regulating inflammation and supporting overall health. Sleep deprivation and poor sleep quality can disrupt the body's immune function and increase levels of inflammatory markers.

Aim for 7-9 hours of uninterrupted sleep each night and establish a consistent sleep schedule by going to bed and waking up at the same time every day.

Create a relaxing bedtime routine to signal to your body that it's time to wind down, such as taking a warm bath, reading a book, or practicing relaxation techniques.

Create a sleep-friendly environment by keeping your bedroom cool, dark, and quiet, and avoiding electronic devices and screens before bedtime.

By incorporating regular exercise, effective stress management techniques, and prioritizing quality sleep into your lifestyle, you can help reduce inflammation in the body and promote optimal health and wellbeing. Making these lifestyle changes can have a positive impact on your overall health and may help reduce the risk of chronic inflammatory conditions.

The role of exercise in combating inflammation

Exercise plays a crucial role in combating inflammation in the body through various mechanisms:

Reduction of Adipose Tissue: Regular exercise helps reduce excess adipose tissue (body fat), particularly visceral fat, which is associated with increased inflammation. By promoting weight loss and maintaining a healthy body composition, exercise can help decrease inflammation levels in the body.

Improvement of Insulin Sensitivity: Exercise enhances insulin sensitivity, allowing cells to more efficiently take up glucose from the bloodstream. Improved insulin sensitivity reduces the production of pro-inflammatory cytokines, which are elevated in insulin-resistant states and contribute to chronic inflammation.

Modulation of the Immune System: Exercise exerts a dual effect on the immune system, promoting a balanced inflammatory response. Acute bouts of exercise can trigger a temporary increase in inflammatory markers as part of the body's normal response to physical exertion. However, regular exercise also leads to adaptations that enhance immune function and reduce chronic low-grade inflammation over time.

Anti-inflammatory Effects of Muscle Contractions: Exercise-induced muscle contractions release myokines, which are cytokines produced by skeletal muscle fibers. Myokines have anti-inflammatory properties and help regulate immune function. For example, interleukin-6 (IL-

6) released during exercise has both pro-inflammatory and anti-inflammatory effects, depending on the context.

Enhancement of Endogenous Antioxidant Defense: Exercise promotes the production of endogenous antioxidants, such as superoxide dismutase (SOD) and glutathione, which help neutralize reactive oxygen species (ROS) and reduce oxidative stress-induced inflammation.

Improvement of Gut Health: Exercise has been shown to modulate the gut microbiota composition, promoting a healthier balance of beneficial bacteria. A healthy gut microbiome is associated with reduced inflammation and improved immune function.

Overall, regular exercise contributes to a state of systemic anti-inflammation by promoting metabolic health, modulating the immune response, and enhancing endogenous antioxidant defenses. By incorporating regular physical activity into your routine, you can help combat inflammation and reduce the risk of chronic inflammatory conditions.

Stress-reducing techniques for inflammation management

Reducing stress is essential for managing inflammation and promoting overall health and wellbeing. Here are some stress-reducing techniques that can help manage inflammation:

Deep Breathing Exercises: Practice deep breathing exercises to activate the body's relaxation response and reduce stress. Try diaphragmatic breathing, where you inhale deeply through your nose, allowing your belly to expand, and exhale slowly through your mouth, focusing on releasing tension from your body.

Mindfulness Meditation: Engage in mindfulness meditation practices to cultivate present-moment awareness and reduce stress. Set aside time each day to practice mindfulness meditation, focusing on your breath, bodily sensations, thoughts, and emotions without judgment.

Progressive Muscle Relaxation: Practice progressive muscle relaxation techniques to release tension and promote relaxation throughout your body. Start by tensing and then relaxing each muscle group sequentially, starting from your toes and working your way up to your head.

Yoga: Incorporate yoga into your routine to promote relaxation, flexibility, and stress reduction. Choose gentle yoga sequences that focus on deep breathing, stretching, and mindfulness to calm the mind and body.

Tai Chi: Consider practicing tai chi, a gentle form of martial arts that combines slow, flowing movements with deep breathing and meditation. Tai chi has been shown to reduce stress, improve balance, and promote overall wellbeing.

Nature Walks: Spend time outdoors in nature to reduce stress and promote relaxation. Take leisurely walks in natural settings such as parks, forests, or beaches, and immerse yourself in the sights, sounds, and smells of the natural world.

Creative Expression: Engage in creative activities such as painting, drawing, writing, or playing music to express yourself and relieve stress. Creative expression can serve as a form of self-care and provide a therapeutic outlet for emotions.

Social Support: Connect with friends, family members, or support groups to share your feelings, experiences, and concerns. Social support can help buffer the effects of stress and promote resilience in challenging times.

Limiting Screen Time: Reduce your exposure to electronic devices and screens, especially before bedtime, to promote relaxation and improve sleep quality. Set boundaries around screen time and prioritize activities that help you unwind and relax.

Healthy Lifestyle Habits: Maintain a balanced diet, get regular exercise, prioritize quality sleep, and practice self-care activities such as massage, hot baths, or aromatherapy to support overall wellbeing and reduce stress levels.

Incorporating these stress-reducing techniques into your daily routine can help manage inflammation, improve resilience to stress, and promote a greater sense of calm and balance in your life. Experiment with different techniques to find what works best for you, and prioritize self-care as an essential component of your inflammation management strategy.

Importance of quality sleep for inflammation control

Quality sleep plays a crucial role in inflammation control and overall health. Here are some reasons why quality sleep is important for managing inflammation:

Regulation of Inflammatory Pathways: Adequate sleep helps regulate the body's inflammatory pathways, preventing excessive inflammation. During sleep, the body produces anti-inflammatory cytokines and suppresses pro-inflammatory cytokines, maintaining a balanced inflammatory response.

Reduction of Systemic Inflammation: Chronic sleep deprivation or poor sleep quality can lead to increased levels of inflammatory markers in the body, such as C-reactive protein (CRP), interleukin-6 (IL-6), and tumor necrosis factor-alpha (TNF-alpha). Prolonged elevation of these inflammatory markers is associated with various inflammatory conditions, including cardiovascular disease, diabetes, and autoimmune disorders.

Immune Function: Quality sleep is essential for optimal immune function, as it supports the body's ability to fight off infections and pathogens. Sleep deprivation compromises the immune system, making individuals more susceptible to infections and increasing inflammation as a result of immune dysregulation.

Regulation of Stress Response: Adequate sleep helps regulate the body's stress response and reduces levels of stress hormones such as cortisol. Chronic stress and elevated cortisol levels can contribute to inflammation and exacerbate inflammatory conditions.

Gut Health: Sleep plays a role in maintaining a healthy gut microbiome, which is essential for regulating inflammation in the body. Disruptions in sleep patterns can alter the composition of the gut microbiota, leading to dysbiosis and increased inflammation.

Metabolic Health: Quality sleep is important for metabolic health, including glucose metabolism and insulin sensitivity. Poor sleep can disrupt metabolic processes, leading to insulin resistance and increased inflammation, which are risk factors for type 2 diabetes and obesity.

Brain Health: Sleep is essential for cognitive function, memory consolidation, and emotional regulation. Chronic sleep deprivation is associated with cognitive impairment, mood disturbances, and increased inflammation in the brain, which may contribute to neurodegenerative diseases such as Alzheimer's disease.

Overall, prioritizing quality sleep is essential for inflammation control and promoting overall health and wellbeing. Aim for 7-9 hours of uninterrupted sleep each night, establish a consistent sleep schedule, create a relaxing bedtime routine, and create a sleep-friendly environment to support optimal sleep quality and inflammation management.

SUPPLEMENTS AND HERBS TO SUPPORT AN ANTI-INFLAMMATORY LIFESTYLE

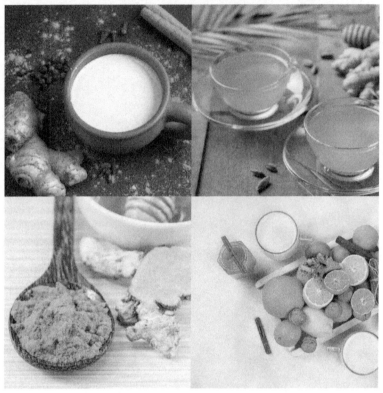

Several supplements and herbs have been studied for their potential anti-inflammatory properties and may support an anti-inflammatory lifestyle when incorporated into a balanced diet and lifestyle. Here are some examples:

Omega-3 Fatty Acids: Omega-3 fatty acids, found in fatty fish like salmon, as well as fish oil supplements, are well-known for their anti-inflammatory effects. They can help reduce inflammation in the body and are beneficial for overall health.

Turmeric/Curcumin: Turmeric contains curcumin, a compound with potent anti-inflammatory and antioxidant properties. Curcumin supplements may help reduce inflammation and alleviate symptoms of inflammatory conditions like arthritis and inflammatory bowel disease.

Ginger: Ginger contains gingerol, a bioactive compound with anti-inflammatory and analgesic properties. Ginger supplements may help reduce inflammation and alleviate pain associated with inflammatory conditions.

Green Tea Extract: Green tea contains polyphenols, such as epigallocatechin gallate (EGCG), which have anti-inflammatory and antioxidant properties. Green tea extract supplements may help reduce inflammation and support overall health.

Resveratrol: Resveratrol is a polyphenol found in red wine, grapes, and berries, known for its anti-inflammatory and antioxidant effects. Resveratrol supplements may help reduce inflammation and protect against chronic diseases.

Quercetin: Quercetin is a flavonoid found in fruits, vegetables, and herbs, known for its anti-inflammatory and immune-modulating effects. Quercetin supplements may help reduce inflammation and support immune health.

Boswellia: Boswellia, also known as Indian frankincense, contains boswellic acids, which have anti-inflammatory properties. Boswellia supplements may help reduce inflammation and alleviate symptoms of inflammatory conditions like osteoarthritis.

Bromelain: Bromelain is an enzyme found in pineapple stems, known for its anti-inflammatory and digestive benefits. Bromelain supplements may help reduce inflammation and promote digestion.

Probiotics: Probiotics are beneficial bacteria that support gut health and immune function. Certain strains of probiotics have been shown to have anti-inflammatory effects and may help reduce inflammation in the body.

Vitamin D: Vitamin D deficiency has been associated with increased inflammation and a higher risk of chronic diseases. Vitamin D supplements may help reduce inflammation and support immune function.

It's important to consult with a healthcare professional before starting any new supplements, especially if you have underlying health conditions or are taking medications, to ensure they are safe and appropriate for you. Additionally, supplements should complement a healthy diet and lifestyle, not replace it. Incorporating a variety of nutrient-rich foods, regular exercise, stress management techniques, and quality sleep is essential for supporting an anti-inflammatory lifestyle.

Supplements that may help reduce inflammation

Here are some supplements that may help reduce inflammation:

Curcumin: Curcumin is the active compound found in turmeric, a spice known for its anti-inflammatory and antioxidant properties. Curcumin supplements may help reduce inflammation and alleviate symptoms of inflammatory conditions such as arthritis and inflammatory bowel disease.

Ginger: Ginger contains bioactive compounds called gingerols, which have anti-inflammatory and analgesic effects. Ginger supplements may help reduce inflammation and alleviate pain associated with inflammatory conditions.

Boswellia: Boswellia, also known as Indian frankincense, contains boswellic acids, which have been shown to have anti-inflammatory properties. Boswellia supplements may help reduce inflammation and alleviate symptoms of conditions like osteoarthritis and rheumatoid arthritis.

Quercetin: Quercetin is a flavonoid with antioxidant and anti-inflammatory properties found in foods like onions, apples, and berries. Quercetin supplements may help reduce inflammation and support immune health.

Green Tea Extract: Green tea contains polyphenols, such as epigallocatechin gallate (EGCG), which have anti-inflammatory and antioxidant effects. Green tea extract supplements may help reduce inflammation and support overall health.

Resveratrol: Resveratrol is a polyphenol found in grapes, red wine, and berries, known for its anti-inflammatory and antioxidant properties. Resveratrol supplements may help reduce inflammation and protect against chronic diseases.

Probiotics: Probiotics are beneficial bacteria that support gut health and immune function. Certain strains of probiotics have been shown to have anti-inflammatory effects and may help reduce inflammation in the body.

Vitamin D: Vitamin D deficiency has been associated with increased inflammation and a higher risk of chronic diseases. Vitamin D supplements may help reduce inflammation and support immune function.

Before starting any new supplement regimen, it's essential to consult with a healthcare professional, especially if you have underlying health conditions or are taking medications. They can provide personalized recommendations based on your individual needs and help ensure that supplements are safe and appropriate for you. Additionally, supplements should complement a healthy diet and lifestyle, not replace it.

Herbal remedies and spices with anti-inflammatory properties

Here are some herbal remedies and spices with anti-inflammatory properties:

Cinnamon: Cinnamon contains antioxidants and anti-inflammatory compounds that may help reduce inflammation in the body. It has been studied for its potential benefits in managing conditions like diabetes and inflammatory bowel disease.

Cloves: Cloves are rich in antioxidants and have anti-inflammatory properties that may help reduce inflammation and promote overall health. Clove oil has been used topically to alleviate pain and inflammation in conditions like toothaches and arthritis.

Rosemary: Rosemary contains rosmarinic acid, a compound with anti-inflammatory and antioxidant effects. It has been studied for its potential benefits in reducing inflammation and supporting brain health.

Oregano: Oregano contains carvacrol and other compounds with anti-inflammatory properties. It has been used traditionally to reduce inflammation and alleviate symptoms of conditions like respiratory infections and arthritis.

Garlic: Garlic contains sulfur compounds with anti-inflammatory and immune-modulating effects. It has been studied for its potential benefits in reducing inflammation and supporting cardiovascular health.

Chili Peppers: Chili peppers contain capsaicin, a compound with anti-inflammatory and pain-relieving properties. Capsaicin has been studied for its potential benefits in reducing inflammation and alleviating symptoms of conditions like arthritis and neuropathic pain.

Black Pepper: Black pepper contains piperine, a compound that enhances the bioavailability of curcumin from turmeric. Combining black pepper with turmeric can enhance the anti-inflammatory effects of curcumin.

Green Tea: Green tea contains polyphenols, such as epigallocatechin gallate (EGCG), which have anti-inflammatory and antioxidant effects. Drinking green tea regularly may help reduce inflammation and support overall health.

Incorporating these herbs and spices into your diet can help reduce inflammation and promote overall health. They can be added to various dishes, teas, or taken as supplements, but it's essential to consult with a healthcare professional before starting any new herbal regimen, especially if you have underlying health conditions or are taking medications.

Guidelines for supplement use and safety

When considering supplement use, it's essential to follow guidelines for safety and efficacy. Here are some general guidelines to keep in mind:

Consult with a Healthcare Professional: Before starting any new supplement regimen, consult with a healthcare professional, such as a doctor or registered dietitian. They can provide personalized recommendations based on your individual health status, medications, and specific needs.

Choose Quality Products: Select supplements from reputable brands that adhere to Good Manufacturing Practices (GMP) and have undergone third-party testing for purity and potency. Look for certifications from organizations like NSF International, USP, or ConsumerLab.com.

Read Labels Carefully: Pay attention to the ingredients list, dosage instructions, and potential allergens or additives in the supplement. Follow the recommended dosage and do not exceed the recommended intake unless advised by a healthcare professional.

Consider Form and Absorption: Choose supplements in forms that are well-absorbed and bioavailable, such as capsules, softgels, or liquid formulations. Some nutrients are better absorbed when taken with food or in combination with other nutrients (e.g., fat-soluble vitamins like vitamin D with a meal containing fat).

Be Cautious of Claims: Be skeptical of supplements that make exaggerated or unsupported claims about their efficacy or health benefits. Look for scientific evidence and research studies supporting the use of the supplement for specific health conditions.

Monitor for Side Effects: Pay attention to how your body responds to supplements and monitor for any adverse reactions or side effects. Discontinue use and consult with a healthcare professional if you experience any negative symptoms.

Avoid Mega-Dosing: Avoid mega-dosing or taking excessive amounts of supplements, as this can increase the risk of adverse effects and toxicity. Stick to recommended dosages and consider obtaining nutrients from food sources whenever possible.

Be Patient: It may take time to see the effects of supplements, particularly for chronic health conditions. Be patient and consistent with your supplement regimen, and give your body time to respond to the nutrients.

Consider Interactions: Be aware of potential interactions between supplements and medications or other supplements you may be taking. Certain supplements can interact with medications or exacerbate underlying health conditions, so it's essential to disclose all supplements to your healthcare provider.

Integrate with a Healthy Lifestyle: Supplements should complement a healthy diet and lifestyle, not replace it. Focus on consuming a balanced diet rich in whole foods, getting regular exercise, managing stress, and prioritizing quality sleep for optimal health and wellbeing.

By following these guidelines, you can make informed choices about supplement use and maximize the potential benefits while minimizing the risks. Remember that supplements are meant to supplement, not substitute, a healthy lifestyle and should be used as part of a comprehensive approach to health and wellness.

NAVIGATING SOCIAL SITUATIONS AND EATING OUT

Navigating social situations and eating out while following an anti-inflammatory lifestyle can be challenging but manageable with some planning and strategies. Here are some tips to help you make healthier choices and stick to your anti-inflammatory diet when dining out:

Plan Ahead: Before going out to eat, research the restaurant's menu online if possible. Look for options that align with your anti-inflammatory diet, such as grilled fish or chicken, salads with lots of vegetables, and side dishes like steamed vegetables or quinoa.

Communicate Your Dietary Needs: Don't hesitate to communicate your dietary preferences and restrictions to the server or restaurant staff. Ask questions about ingredients, preparation methods, and possible substitutions to ensure your meal meets your dietary requirements.

Choose Wisely: Opt for dishes that are rich in fruits, vegetables, whole grains, lean proteins, and healthy fats. Avoid fried foods, processed meats, refined carbohydrates, and dishes with added sugars and excessive amounts of salt.

Customize Your Order: Don't be afraid to customize your order to suit your dietary needs. Ask for sauces, dressings, and condiments on the side, request grilled or steamed options instead of fried, and substitute vegetables or a side salad for fries or other less healthy sides.

Watch Portion Sizes: Be mindful of portion sizes, as restaurant servings tend to be larger than what you might eat at home. Consider sharing an entree with a friend or ordering a smaller portion if available. Listen to your body's hunger and fullness cues and stop eating when you're satisfied.

Limit Alcohol Consumption: Alcohol can be inflammatory, so limit your intake or choose healthier options like red wine or cocktails made with fresh ingredients and minimal added sugars. Stay hydrated by drinking plenty of water throughout your meal.

Be Flexible: Remember that it's okay to be flexible with your diet on occasion, especially in social settings. Focus on making the best choices available to you, but don't stress too much if you can't adhere perfectly to your anti-inflammatory diet.

Practice Mindful Eating: Slow down and savor each bite, paying attention to the flavors, textures, and sensations of the food. Eating mindfully can help you enjoy your meal more fully and prevent overeating.

Bring Your Own: If you're attending a gathering or event where food will be served, consider bringing a dish or two that align with your anti-inflammatory diet. This ensures you'll have healthy options to enjoy and share with others.

Focus on Enjoyment: Ultimately, dining out should be an enjoyable experience. Focus on the social aspect of the meal, enjoy the company of friends and loved ones, and don't stress too much about sticking rigidly to your diet.

By planning ahead, communicating your dietary needs, making smart choices, and practicing mindfulness, you can successfully navigate social situations and eating out while following an anti-inflammatory lifestyle. Remember to be flexible, enjoy your meals, and prioritize overall health and wellbeing.

Tips for dining out while following an anti-inflammatory diet

Navigating dining out while following an anti-inflammatory diet can be challenging, but with some preparation and mindfulness, you can make healthier choices. Here are some tips to help you dine out while sticking to your anti-inflammatory diet:

Research Restaurants: Before choosing a restaurant, look up their menu online to see if they offer options that align with your anti-inflammatory diet. Many restaurants now include dietary information or labels for gluten-free, vegetarian, or healthier choices.

Choose Simple Preparations: Look for dishes that are grilled, baked, steamed, or roasted, as these cooking methods typically involve less added fat and are lower in calories. Avoid dishes that are fried, breaded, or heavily sauced, as they may contain hidden inflammatory ingredients.

Focus on Vegetables: Make vegetables the star of your meal by choosing dishes that feature a variety of colorful vegetables. Salads, vegetable stir-fries, grilled vegetable platters, and vegetable-based soups are excellent choices that are rich in anti-inflammatory nutrients.

Opt for Lean Proteins: Choose lean protein sources such as grilled chicken, fish, tofu, or legumes to accompany your meal. These options are lower in saturated fat and calories compared to red meats and processed meats, which can contribute to inflammation.

Be Wary of Sauces and Dressings: Many restaurant sauces, dressings, and marinades contain added sugars, unhealthy fats, and preservatives that can contribute to inflammation. Ask for sauces and dressings on the side, or inquire about healthier options such as olive oil and vinegar or fresh herbs.

Customize Your Order: Don't hesitate to ask for substitutions or modifications to suit your dietary needs. Most restaurants are willing to accommodate special requests, such as substituting steamed vegetables for fries or serving sauces on the side.

Limit Refined Carbohydrates: Be mindful of refined carbohydrates such as white bread, pasta, rice, and potatoes, as they can cause spikes in blood sugar and contribute to inflammation. Choose whole grain or alternative grain options whenever possible.

Hydrate Wisely: Opt for water, herbal tea, or unsweetened beverages instead of sugary sodas, juices, or alcoholic drinks. Staying hydrated with water helps flush toxins from the body and supports overall health.

Practice Portion Control: Restaurant portions tend to be larger than what you might eat at home, so practice portion control by sharing an entree with a friend, ordering a smaller portion, or saving half of your meal for later.

Listen to Your Body: Pay attention to how different foods make you feel and adjust your choices accordingly. Choose foods that leave you feeling energized, satisfied, and free of digestive discomfort.

By following these tips and being mindful of your choices, you can enjoy dining out while still adhering to your anti-inflammatory diet and supporting your overall health and wellbeing.

Strategies for social gatherings and parties

Attending social gatherings and parties while following an anti-inflammatory diet may require some planning and strategies to navigate food options and stick to your dietary goals. Here are some strategies to help you enjoy social events while staying true to your anti-inflammatory lifestyle:

Eat Before You Go: Have a nutritious snack or meal before heading to the event to help curb hunger and prevent overeating unhealthy foods once you arrive. This will also help you make better choices when faced with tempting treats.

Bring Your Own Dish: Offer to bring a dish or two that align with your anti-inflammatory diet to share with others. This ensures that you'll have at least one healthy option to enjoy and introduces others to delicious and nutritious alternatives.

Scan the Buffet or Spread: Before filling your plate, take a quick scan of the food options available. Look for dishes that are likely to be lower in inflammatory ingredients, such as salads, vegetable platters, grilled proteins, and fruit trays.

Fill Up on Vegetables: Load up your plate with colorful vegetables, which are rich in anti-inflammatory nutrients and fiber. Choose raw or lightly cooked vegetables without heavy sauces or dressings.

Choose Lean Proteins: Opt for lean protein sources such as grilled chicken, fish, tofu, or legumes to help keep you satisfied and provide essential nutrients without contributing to inflammation.

Be Mindful of Portions: Practice portion control by taking smaller portions of higher-calorie or indulgent foods and larger portions of healthier options like vegetables and lean proteins. Remember to listen to your body's hunger and fullness cues.

Watch Your Beverages: Be mindful of your beverage choices, as sugary cocktails, sodas, and alcoholic drinks can contribute to inflammation. Opt for water, herbal tea, or sparkling water with a splash of fruit juice as a healthier alternative.

Limit Alcohol Intake: If you choose to drink alcohol, do so in moderation, as excessive alcohol consumption can increase inflammation in the body. Stick to one or two drinks and alternate with water to stay hydrated.

Practice the 80/20 Rule: Allow yourself some flexibility and enjoyment by following the 80/20 rule, where you aim to make healthy choices 80% of the time and allow for occasional indulgences 20% of the time. This approach can help you maintain balance and prevent feelings of deprivation.

Focus on Socializing: Remember that social gatherings are about more than just food. Focus on enjoying the company of friends and loved ones, engaging in conversation, and participating in activities rather than solely focusing on the food available.

By implementing these strategies and being mindful of your choices, you can navigate social gatherings and parties while still adhering to your anti-inflammatory diet and supporting your health goals.

How to communicate your dietary needs to others

Communicating your dietary needs to others can be done effectively and respectfully using the following strategies:

Be Clear and Specific: Clearly communicate your dietary preferences and restrictions to others. Use specific terms and language to describe what you can and cannot eat, including any allergies, intolerances, or dietary choices (e.g., gluten-free, dairy-free, vegetarian, vegan).

Provide Information: Offer information about your dietary needs and the reasons behind them, if necessary. Explain that you follow a specific diet for health reasons, personal preferences, religious beliefs, or ethical considerations. Providing context can help others understand and respect your choices.

Be Proactive: Take the initiative to communicate your dietary needs in advance, especially when attending events or gatherings where food will be served. Reach out to the host or organizer to discuss menu options and inquire about accommodations if needed.

Ask Questions: Don't hesitate to ask questions about ingredients, preparation methods, and possible substitutions when dining out or attending events. Seek clarification to ensure that the food meets your dietary requirements and preferences.

Express Appreciation: Express gratitude to others for accommodating your dietary needs and making an effort to provide suitable options. Acknowledge their efforts and show appreciation for their understanding and support.

Offer to Bring Your Own: Offer to bring a dish or two that align with your dietary needs to share with others. This ensures that you'll have something to eat that meets your requirements and takes the pressure off the host to accommodate your needs entirely.

Be Flexible: Be flexible and open-minded when communicating your dietary needs to others. Understand that not everyone may be familiar with your specific dietary preferences or restrictions, and be willing to compromise or make adjustments when necessary.

Educate and Advocate: Take the opportunity to educate others about your dietary needs and advocate for yourself when needed. Share information about your diet, provide resources or recommendations for suitable options, and advocate for inclusive menus and accommodations.

Set Boundaries: Set boundaries and assertively communicate your needs when faced with pressure or pushback from others. Respectfully decline foods that do not align with your dietary requirements and assert your right to make choices that support your health and wellbeing.

Lead by Example: Lead by example and demonstrate the benefits of your dietary choices through your actions and behaviors. Show others that eating healthily can be enjoyable, delicious, and fulfilling, and inspire them to make healthier choices themselves.

By using these strategies to communicate your dietary needs effectively, you can ensure that others understand and respect your preferences while supporting your health and wellbeing.

OVERCOMING CHALLENGES AND MAINTAINING LONG-TERM SUCCESS

Maintaining long-term success with an anti-inflammatory lifestyle requires overcoming various challenges and adopting sustainable habits. Here are some strategies to help you overcome challenges and maintain your progress:

Set Realistic Goals: Set realistic and achievable goals for yourself, whether it's incorporating more anti-inflammatory foods into your diet, increasing physical activity, or managing stress more effectively. Break larger goals into smaller, manageable steps to make progress more attainable.

Educate Yourself: Continuously educate yourself about the principles of anti-inflammatory living, including the benefits of specific foods, lifestyle factors, and stress management techniques. Stay informed about the latest research and evidence-based recommendations to support your journey.

Build a Support Network: Surround yourself with a supportive network of friends, family members, or online communities who share similar health goals and values. Having a support system can provide encouragement, accountability, and motivation during challenging times.

Practice Self-Compassion: Be kind to yourself and practice self-compassion as you navigate your anti-inflammatory lifestyle journey. Recognize that setbacks and obstacles are a normal part of the process and focus on progress rather than perfection.

Plan and Prepare: Plan ahead and prepare healthy meals and snacks in advance to avoid relying on convenience foods or making impulsive choices. Stock your pantry with anti-inflammatory staples, batch cook meals, and pack nutritious snacks for when you're on the go.

Stay Flexible: Be flexible and adaptable in your approach to anti-inflammatory living, especially when faced with unexpected challenges or changes in routine. Learn to navigate social situations, travel, and dining out while still making choices that align with your goals.

Practice Mindful Eating: Practice mindful eating by paying attention to hunger and fullness cues, savoring the flavors and textures of your food, and eating slowly and attentively. Mindful eating can help prevent overeating, reduce stress-related eating, and enhance enjoyment of meals.

Stay Active: Incorporate regular physical activity into your routine to support overall health and reduce inflammation in the body. Find activities you enjoy, whether it's walking, cycling, yoga, or dancing, and make movement a regular part of your lifestyle.

Manage Stress: Implement stress management techniques such as deep breathing exercises, meditation, yoga, or spending time in nature to reduce stress levels and promote relaxation. Chronic stress can contribute to inflammation, so prioritizing stress reduction is essential for long-term success.

Celebrate Progress: Celebrate your successes and milestones along the way, no matter how small they may seem. Acknowledge your efforts and achievements, and use them as motivation to keep moving forward on your anti-inflammatory journey.

By implementing these strategies and cultivating a holistic approach to anti-inflammatory living, you can overcome challenges and maintain long-term success in supporting your health and wellbeing. Remember that consistency, perseverance, and self-care are key components of sustainable lifestyle change.

Common obstacles to sticking to an anti-inflammatory lifestyle

Sticking to an anti-inflammatory lifestyle can be challenging due to various obstacles. Some common obstacles include:

Limited Food Options: Finding suitable food options that align with an anti-inflammatory diet can be difficult, especially when dining out or traveling. Limited access to fresh, whole foods and reliance on processed or convenience foods can hinder adherence to the diet.

Social Pressure: Social gatherings, parties, and events often revolve around food, making it challenging to stick to an anti-inflammatory diet when faced with peer pressure or temptations. Well-meaning friends or family members may also question or criticize dietary choices, adding to the pressure.

Time Constraints: Busy schedules and hectic lifestyles can make it challenging to prioritize meal planning, grocery shopping, and cooking nutritious meals at home. Convenience foods and fast food options may seem more appealing when time is limited.

Emotional Eating: Emotional factors such as stress, boredom, sadness, or loneliness can trigger cravings for unhealthy, inflammatory foods as a coping mechanism. Emotional eating habits can undermine efforts to stick to an anti-inflammatory diet and lead to overeating or binge eating.

Food Cravings: Cravings for sugary, salty, or processed foods can be difficult to resist, especially if these foods were previously staples in your diet. Cravings can be triggered by hormonal fluctuations, nutrient deficiencies, or environmental cues, making them hard to overcome.

Lack of Support: Lack of support from friends, family members, or healthcare providers can make it challenging to maintain motivation and adherence to an anti-inflammatory lifestyle. Negative attitudes, skepticism, or lack of understanding about the benefits of the diet can undermine efforts to stick to it.

Expense: Eating a nutrient-dense, anti-inflammatory diet that includes plenty of fresh fruits, vegetables, and lean proteins can be more expensive than a diet based on processed or convenience foods. Cost barriers may limit access to healthy food options for some individuals.

Food Sensitivities: Undiagnosed food sensitivities or allergies can make it difficult to identify inflammatory triggers in the diet and may lead to symptoms such as digestive issues, fatigue, headaches, or joint pain.

Eliminating inflammatory foods without proper guidance or testing can be challenging and may result in nutrient deficiencies.

Cultural or Dietary Preferences: Cultural or dietary preferences may clash with the principles of an anti-inflammatory diet, making it challenging to stick to the guidelines. Traditional or cultural foods may be high in inflammatory ingredients or prepared in ways that are incompatible with the diet.

Lack of Education: Limited knowledge or understanding of the principles of anti-inflammatory eating, including which foods to include or avoid, can hinder adherence to the diet. Without proper education or guidance, individuals may struggle to make informed choices and maintain consistency.

Overcoming these obstacles requires a combination of education, planning, support, and self-awareness. By addressing these challenges proactively and developing strategies to overcome them, individuals can successfully stick to an anti-inflammatory lifestyle and reap the health benefits over the long term.

Strategies for staying motivated and on track

Staying motivated and on track with an anti-inflammatory lifestyle requires commitment, consistency, and a proactive approach. Here are some strategies to help you stay motivated and maintain your progress:

Set Clear Goals: Define specific, measurable, and achievable goals for yourself related to your anti-inflammatory lifestyle, such as incorporating more fruits and vegetables into your diet, exercising regularly, or reducing stress levels. Write down your goals and revisit them regularly to stay focused and motivated.

Educate Yourself: Continuously educate yourself about the benefits of an anti-inflammatory lifestyle and the impact of nutrition, exercise, sleep, and stress management on inflammation and overall health. Stay informed about the latest research and evidence-based recommendations to reinforce your commitment to your goals.

Find Your Why: Identify your reasons for adopting an anti-inflammatory lifestyle and remind yourself of them regularly. Whether it's improving your health, managing chronic conditions, increasing energy levels, or enhancing overall wellbeing, connecting with your underlying motivations can help sustain your commitment.

Track Your Progress: Keep track of your progress toward your goals using a journal, planner, app, or tracking tool. Monitor your food intake, physical activity, sleep patterns, and stress levels, as well as any changes in symptoms or health outcomes. Celebrate your successes and milestones along the way to stay motivated.

Create Accountability: Share your goals and progress with a friend, family member, or health coach who can provide support, encouragement, and accountability. Consider joining a support group or online community of like-minded individuals who share similar health goals and challenges.

Plan and Prepare: Plan your meals, snacks, and exercise sessions in advance to avoid relying on convenience foods or making impulsive choices. Stock your pantry with anti-inflammatory staples, batch cook meals, and schedule regular physical activity sessions to make healthy habits more manageable.

Practice Self-Care: Prioritize self-care activities that support your physical, mental, and emotional wellbeing, such as getting adequate sleep, practicing relaxation techniques, spending time outdoors, and engaging in hobbies or activities you enjoy. Taking care of yourself holistically can boost motivation and resilience.

Focus on Progress, Not Perfection: Embrace the concept of progress over perfection and recognize that small, consistent changes add up over time. Celebrate your efforts and achievements, even if they're not always perfect, and use setbacks or challenges as opportunities for growth and learning.

Visualize Success: Use visualization techniques to imagine yourself achieving your goals and living your ideal anti-inflammatory lifestyle. Visualize how you will look, feel, and function when you reach your desired outcomes, and use these mental images as motivation to keep moving forward.

Stay Flexible and Adapt: Be flexible and adaptable in your approach to an anti-inflammatory lifestyle, especially when faced with unexpected challenges or changes in circumstances. Learn to adjust your plans, make modifications as needed, and stay resilient in the face of setbacks.

By implementing these strategies and staying committed to your goals, you can stay motivated and on track with your anti-inflammatory lifestyle, leading to improved health and wellbeing over the long term.

CONCLUSION: EMBRACING YOUR NEW ANTI-INFLAMMATORY LIFESTYLE

In conclusion, embracing your new anti-inflammatory lifestyle is a journey of self-discovery, empowerment, and transformation. By prioritizing your health and wellbeing, you've taken proactive steps to reduce inflammation, improve vitality, and enhance your overall quality of life. Throughout this journey, you've learned valuable insights, strategies, and skills that will serve you well in the pursuit of optimal health and longevity.

As you continue to incorporate anti-inflammatory principles into your daily routine, remember to approach this lifestyle with compassion, curiosity, and flexibility. Embrace the process of learning and experimentation, knowing that every choice you make contributes to your wellbeing in meaningful ways. Celebrate your successes and milestones along the way, recognizing the progress you've made and the positive changes you've experienced.

Moving forward, stay committed to your goals, but also remain open to adaptation and growth. Listen to your body's cues, honor your unique needs and preferences, and trust in your ability to make empowered choices that support your health and happiness. Surround yourself with a supportive network of friends, family members, and healthcare professionals who champion your journey and encourage your success.

Above all, remember that your anti-inflammatory lifestyle is not just about what you eat or how you move—it's about cultivating a holistic approach to health that nourishes your body, mind, and spirit. By nourishing yourself with wholesome foods, engaging in regular physical activity, managing stress effectively, prioritizing quality sleep, and fostering meaningful connections, you can create a life filled with vitality, resilience, and joy.

As you embrace your new anti-inflammatory lifestyle, may you find fulfillment, inspiration, and empowerment in every moment. Here's to your health, happiness, and wellbeing, today and always.

Reflecting on your journey

Reflecting on your anti-inflammatory journey is an important practice that allows you to recognize your progress, learn from your experiences, and gain insight into your health and wellness. Take a moment to reflect on your journey by considering the following questions:

What motivated you to adopt an anti-inflammatory lifestyle?

Reflect on the reasons behind your decision to prioritize your health and wellbeing. Consider any health concerns, goals, or personal values that inspired you to make changes.

What changes have you noticed since implementing anti-inflammatory principles into your life?

Take stock of the positive changes you've experienced, both physically and emotionally. Consider improvements in energy levels, digestion, sleep quality, mood, and overall vitality.

What challenges have you encountered along the way? How did you overcome them?

Reflect on any obstacles or setbacks you've faced during your journey. Consider the strategies, resources, or support systems that helped you navigate challenges and stay on track.

What have you learned about yourself and your relationship with food, exercise, and self-care?

Explore any insights or revelations you've gained about your habits, preferences, and behaviors related to food, movement, stress management, and self-care. Consider how these insights have informed your approach to health and wellness.

How have your priorities or perspectives shifted since embracing an anti-inflammatory lifestyle?

Consider any shifts in mindset, values, or priorities that have occurred as a result of your journey. Reflect on how your relationship with health, food, and self-care has evolved over time.

What accomplishments or milestones are you most proud of?

Celebrate your successes and achievements, no matter how small. Acknowledge the progress you've made and the positive changes you've implemented in your life.

What goals or aspirations do you have for the future of your anti-inflammatory journey?

Look ahead and consider your goals, dreams, and aspirations for continued growth and development. Think about how you can build upon your successes and continue to prioritize your health and wellbeing.

How do you plan to sustain and maintain your anti-inflammatory lifestyle in the long term?

Reflect on strategies for sustaining your progress and staying committed to your goals over the long term.

Consider how you can integrate anti-inflammatory principles into your daily life in a way that feels sustainable and enjoyable.

By reflecting on your anti-inflammatory journey, you can gain valuable insights, cultivate gratitude for your progress, and reaffirm your commitment to your health and wellbeing. Use this opportunity to celebrate your achievements, learn from your experiences, and chart a course for continued growth and success in the future.

Long-term goals for maintaining an anti-inflammatory lifestyle

Setting long-term goals for maintaining an anti-inflammatory lifestyle is essential for sustaining your progress and promoting lasting health and wellbeing. Here are some long-term goals to consider:

Consistent Nutrient-Rich Diet: Aim to consistently follow a nutrient-rich diet that is high in anti-inflammatory foods such as fruits, vegetables, whole grains, lean proteins, and healthy fats. Make it a priority to incorporate a variety of colorful, whole foods into your meals to ensure you're getting a wide range of nutrients and phytochemicals.

Regular Physical Activity: Commit to regular physical activity as part of your anti-inflammatory lifestyle. Set a goal to engage in moderate-intensity exercise, such as brisk walking, swimming, cycling, or yoga, for at least 150 minutes per week, as recommended by health guidelines. Find activities you enjoy and make them a regular part of your routine.

Stress Management: Prioritize stress management techniques to reduce the impact of chronic stress on inflammation and overall health. Incorporate practices such as mindfulness meditation, deep breathing exercises, progressive muscle relaxation, or spending time in nature to promote relaxation and resilience.

Quality Sleep: Focus on optimizing sleep quality and quantity to support inflammation control and overall wellbeing. Aim for 7-9 hours of restful sleep per night and establish a consistent sleep schedule by going to bed and waking up at the same time each day. Create a relaxing bedtime routine and create a sleep-friendly environment to promote restorative sleep.

Healthy Weight Management: Maintain a healthy weight through a balanced diet, regular physical activity, and lifestyle habits that support metabolic health. Set realistic weight management goals based on your individual needs and focus on making sustainable changes to your diet and lifestyle to achieve and maintain a healthy weight over time.

Regular Health Monitoring: Schedule regular health check-ups and screenings with your healthcare provider to monitor your overall health and assess your progress towards your anti-inflammatory goals. Keep track of key health markers such as blood pressure, cholesterol levels, blood sugar levels, and inflammatory markers to stay informed about your health status.

Continued Education: Commit to ongoing education and learning about anti-inflammatory principles, nutrition, exercise, and lifestyle factors that promote health and wellbeing. Stay informed about the latest research and evidence-based recommendations to enhance your knowledge and empower yourself to make informed choices.

Adaptability and Flexibility: Remain adaptable and flexible in your approach to maintaining an anti-inflammatory lifestyle. Recognize that life circumstances may change, and your needs and priorities may evolve over time. Be open to adjusting your goals, strategies, and habits as needed to accommodate changes and challenges.

Cultivate Supportive Relationships: Cultivate supportive relationships with friends, family members, or healthcare professionals who understand and support your anti-inflammatory lifestyle. Surround yourself with individuals who encourage and uplift you on your journey towards better health and wellbeing.

Celebrate Progress: Celebrate your progress and achievements along the way, no matter how small. Acknowledge your efforts and successes, and use them as motivation to continue making positive changes in your life. Take pride in your commitment to maintaining an anti-inflammatory lifestyle and the positive impact it has on your health and wellbeing.

By setting and working towards these long-term goals, you can maintain your anti-inflammatory lifestyle and enjoy the many benefits of improved health, vitality, and longevity over the years to come.

Printed in Great Britain
by Amazon

44765424R00076